Special Praise for
Love in the Land of Dementia

"*Love in the Land of Dementia* is a very moving, but also convincing story. I recommend it as a good read for other caregivers who can be encouraged for their own caregiving journey. It is also important for the rest of us, who should not forget how big the impact of this disease is on people's lives, and how urgently we need to advocate for better care, support, and ultimately finding a cure for Alzheimer's disease and other dementias."

—Marc Wortmann
Executive Director, Alzheimer's Disease International

"This is a story of love and compassion that is deeply personal, as well as giving a voice to so many people with dementia and their families. This book is written with honesty, insight, and humour, and will help society understand what it is like to support someone close with dementia, as well as offering some practical guidance. By humanising dementia, Deborah is reducing the social stigma so the social world around each person with dementia can offer compassion and love instead of judging and labelling. This book represents a personal journey to a new, enlightened paradigm of dementia care."

—Jane Verity
Founder and CEO
Dementia Care Australia

"We have been searching for a text by a family caregiver that we can recommend unreservedly, and now we feel we have found one in *Love in the Land of Dementia* by Deborah Shouse. Whilst never denying the downturns in caring for someone with Alzheimer's, Deborah is intelligent and sensitive enough to notice all sorts of things that bring situations alive, give people hope, and constitute treasurable epiphanies."

—John Killick
Author and Alzheimer's Advocate
Dementia Positive, UK, *The Journal of Dementia Care*

"*Love in the Land of Dementia* is an insightful journey of a daughter as her mother progresses through the stages of Alzheimer's disease. There is wisdom in every anecdote, and Deborah Shouse's unique perspective provides caregivers and family members with hope and meaning."
—Jeffrey M. Burns, MD
Director, Alzheimer and Memory Center
Principal Investigator, Brain Aging Project,
University of Kansas Medical Center

"I have read hundreds of true stories about families dealing with Alzheimer's disease. None was written more wonderfully or truthfully about the grief, guilt, and, yes, grace of caring for someone with this disease. Readers journey with Deborah Shouse in her superbly written tale, finding hope in the loss and even happiness in the new connection."
—LeAnn Thiemann
Coauthor, *Chicken Soup for the Caregiver's Soul*

"Deborah Shouse extends a glimpse of humanity within the very challenging role of Alzheimer's disease and long-term care. Her stories have a message that cannot be conveyed or received in any better way. The stories are beautiful and wrought with genuine compassion."
—Michelle Niedens
Education Director
Alzheimer's Association, Heart of America Chapter

LOVE
in the Land *of*
Dementia

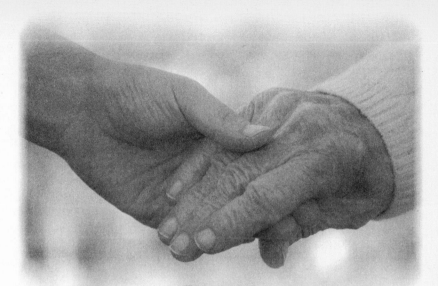

LOVE
in the Land *of*
Dementia

Finding Hope in the Caregiver's Journey

DEBORAH SHOUSE

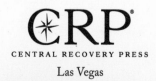

CENTRAL RECOVERY PRESS

Las Vegas

Central Recovery Press (CRP) is committed to publishing exceptional materials addressing addiction treatment, recovery, and behavioral healthcare topics, including original and quality books, audio/visual communications, and web-based new media. Through a diverse selection of titles, we seek to contribute a broad range of unique resources for professionals, recovering individuals and their families, and the general public.

For more information, visit www.centralrecoverypress.com.

Central Recovery Press
3321 N. Buffalo Drive
Las Vegas, NV 89129

18 17 16 15 14 13   1 2 3 4 5

ISBN: 978-1-937612-49-8 (paper)
        978-1-937612-50-4 (e-book)

Publisher's Note: This is a memoir, an inspirational and autobiographical work based on fact recorded to the best of the author's memory. To protect their privacy, the names of some of the people and institutions in this book have been changed, but any facts recounted are historically accurate.

Cover design, illustration, interior design, and layout by
Deb Tremper, Six Penny Graphics

I dedicate this love story to my parents,
Fran and Paul Barnett.

Table of Contents

Foreword

Several years ago, I was a speaker at a national conference on aging, along with thousands of academics and other professionals. After my closing address, an elderly man came down the aisle toward me, pushing his wife in her wheelchair. He had that look in his eye that said, "Listen here, young man, I am coming to talk to you; you stay right where you are." I did.

After a few pleasantries, during which I noticed that his wife was paralyzed, drooling, and clearly in her own reality, the man said, "Isn't she pretty?" I immediately replied, "Yes, sir." He started telling me about how they had been members of their church for fifty-five years, when suddenly his wife coughed, gagging on her saliva. For a moment I thought she was going to die, but her husband calmly removed a handkerchief from his pocket and tenderly cleaned her up. Then he turned to me and said, "I love her very much. I bathe her, I dress her, and I take her everywhere." Then he related how the previous week, his minister had told him that members of his Sunday school class had requested that he not bring his wife to class anymore. The reason? His wife made them uncomfortable. Brimming with anger, the man said, "And what do you think about that, Dr. Oliver?" It was a declaration, not a question.

As he left, I realized that his were the most profound words spoken at the conference. He had said, "The problem is not my wife; it is those people in the Sunday school class." It is you and me. It is those of us who are uncomfortable with frailness, helplessness, dependency, and more. Though our reaction is normal, we are the problem. Ultimately, it is the rest of us who need hope and help. If we can enter the land of dementia with open hearts, minds, and souls, we might just be healed by those who are the object of our love.

Deborah Shouse did enter the land of dementia. This book, *Love in the Land of Dementia,* is a must-read for all of us.

Storytelling is an art, and Deborah Shouse has taken it to a new level. More important, she has opened an album of her life that hits the target with every image and experience that accompanies dementia in general, and Alzheimer's disease in particular.

This book is an extraordinary celebration, yet it also captures the pain, anguish, and sense of hopelessness that people can feel when surrounded and influenced by this disease. Through her stories, Deborah shows us the complex and often inseparable relationship between love and grief. Those of us who have experienced the journey of dementia with a loved one know it can be both a terrifying ordeal and the most meaningful love story of all time.

Responding to dementia requires a strong and loving person who can get out of his or her own skin and enter the loved one's reality. It is not easy, and many will not make it. Deborah made it and can help the rest of us.

Read her story.

David B. Oliver, PhD

Assistant Director, MU Interdisciplinary Center on Aging

Department of Family and Community Medicine, University of Missouri

Recipient of the Outstanding Educator of the Year Award from

the American College of Health Care Administrators

Author of *The Human Factor in Nursing Home Care*

A Note from Deborah

One of the great lessons I've learned from sharing my personal stories is just how connected we caregivers are, no matter where we live. As my life and performance partner Ron and I have traveled, we've offered a performance of my stories from this book when we've visited a new country. After our performance in Istanbul, a man stepped forward, his hat in his hands. Through the Turkish translator, he shyly told me, "My wife has Alzheimer's and I've taken care of her for ten years. Your story is my story."

Our first foreign event was in Dunedin, New Zealand, where we were warmly welcomed by the Alzheimer's Society. After we shared a few personal experiences, a woman came up to me and said, "I really like your accent." She had cared for her husband for years and had continued to volunteer at the society after his death. "These people really understand me," she said.

A year later, Ron and I sat in a cafeteria in San Jose, Costa Rica, waiting to meet the man who would be doing a simultaneous Spanish translation of our performance. As Ron and I sipped tea, we heard a melodious voice say, "Go Jayhawks." It turns out our translator had studied at the University of Kansas, a mere forty minutes away from our home in Kansas City. Like us, he became involved in Alzheimer's through personal experience.

In Florence, Italy, we shared our stories in an eleventh-century church, where the priest told us all, "The Alzheimer's patient is the pupil in God's eye."

We spoke at a Victorian hall in Barnet, England, the very town that my grandfather ran away to as a thirteen-year-old boy so he would not be pressed into the Russian army. We have shared my stories in a Dublin community center and in a conference center in St. Croix. Our two translators in San Juan, Puerto Rico, met each other when visiting their respective spouses in an Alzheimer's facility and fell in love. Having them read with us added an additional layer of emotion to the performance.

Though the language and the venue may have changed, each performance—from the one in Santiago, Chile, to the one in Hiawatha, Kansas—reminded us of how connected all of us are in this journey. Whether the culture was one with care centers and Alzheimer's units or whether home care was the norm, the caregiver's worries, fears, exhaustion, confusion, gratitude, and blessings were much the same. And they still are.

I originally self-published this book, wanting to use all the money it generated as a donation to Alzheimer's programs and research. My goal was to raise $50,000; over the years, using the book as a catalyst, my partner Ron and I have raised more than $80,000 for Alzheimer's. I believe this indicates the growing numbers of people who are affected by this disease, and how much they hunger for support and understanding.

I wrote this book first for myself and then for you—I wanted to share my journey as a caregiver, hoping it could comfort and inspire others. I look forward to hearing from you and learning more about the blessings and lessons you've gleaned from your time with *Love in the Land of Dementia*.

Acknowledgments

So many people helped and encouraged me in the writing of these stories. My life partner Ron Zoglin has read each story many times. My critique partners Andrea Warren and Barbara Bartocci helped me edit and strengthen each essay. Andrea came up with the title for the book. My dear friend Maril Crabtree also helped me edit and shape the stories. Linda Rodriguez, Sally Berneathy, Judith Fertig, Robin Silverman, and Jane Wood helped me hone the collection. Victoria Moran and Sarah Grace Parlak encouraged and inspired me. Pola Firestone helped me with ideas; Mary Beth Gordon and Kirsten McBride assisted with editing and proofreading. Rex and Jane Rogers, endlessly, patiently, helped bring the original manuscript to visual life. Bernadette Stankard connected me to Central Recovery Press and has been a supportive and encouraging guide.

As always, the members of the Kansas City Writer's Group offered encouragement and support. I am so grateful for their energy and their presence. I am also grateful to all the friends and caregivers who have supported our Alzheimer's performances with their presence and given us vital feedback and encouragement.

My family has also helped, inspired, and sustained me. My brother Daniel Barnett lived through these stories with me, as did my daughters, Sarah and Hilee, and my niece and nephews, Helen, Zachary, and Jake. Zachary helped with artistic inspiration. My Aunt Ethel shared stories with me, and my cousins so kindly encouraged me. Ron's brother Bobby and his parents, Mollie and Frank, were always a source of encouragement. One of my mother's dearest friends, Fran, was another source of lovely encouragement. Guy Guber, son of Bel and Max, was a light for me.

Thanks to our area Alzheimer's Association and to Michelle, Debra, Kelly, Clemme, Jeanne, Shannon, and others for all their amazing support and help.

My mother had many wonderful caretakers and I am grateful to all of them for their loving care. Special thanks to Pam, Chris, Patrice, and Deborah, and to Kathy Riggs and her wonderful parents. I am also grateful to the marvelous people with Alzheimer's I met and to that community of patients and families.

Before

"Don't stay out too late," my mother says, handing me her car keys.

"Do you want to wait up for me?" I ask her.

She shrugs. "I won't be able to sleep anyway."

When I left Kansas City to come visit my mother, I was a mature woman. But once I enter my mother's house, I revert to my earliest, most practiced role, that of daughter.

Every mother knows so much more than her daughter. Every mother sees the beauty, the secret hollows, and the lost potential of her daughter. The mother saves these insights like precious unread love letters. She prays that somehow, someday, her daughter will ask her just how much she knows.

I, too, am a mother. I know the exact words that could change my daughters into happier women. And like my own mother, I wait helplessly for them to open their ears to me.

I return to my mother's house before midnight. Though my old friends tried to persuade me to go to just one more jazz club, I felt my mother waiting for me. She opens the door before I even knock.

"I have something to show you," she says. I follow her into the breakfast room.

"Look at this," she says, pointing to a photo of a beautiful woman sitting coquettishly under a tree. Her lipstick is a taunting red, her hair a provocative black.

"This was taken when I was in nurse's training," my mother says. I see her secret smile, her joy in how beautiful she was.

I sit down and study the picture, knowing that when it was taken she had already lost her mother and her first husband; that deep sorrow stretched underneath her beauty. Then my mother spreads more pictures. Me at age five, playing jacks on the front porch. Me and my daughters sitting in a mimosa tree.

"No one can hurt you as much as your own daughter can," my mother says as she hands me another photo, one of my wedding. "I knew you were making a big mistake," she says, jabbing her finger at my ex-husband's picture.

Before, when my mother made remarks like this, I resented it. But on this visit, I listen. I allow the words to soak in. I hear their translation: "I love you. I think of you all the time. You are so important to me." Had she been speaking in a foreign language all these years, so I never noticed the real meaning of her words?

I call home to check on my fifteen-year-old daughter.

"Hi, how are you?" I ask.

"Fine," she answers.

"How was your day?"

"Okay."

I know when she is done talking to me, she will call her friends and they will laugh and chat for hours. I feel like a thirsty woman, wanting too many drops of water.

"Want some coffee, dear?" my mother asks when I get off the phone.

I take the coffee, made the way my mother likes it, too strong. We sit together on the sofa, and she asks me if I eat properly.

I want to answer, "Yes," in a voice as crisp and clipped as my daughter's. I take a deep breath before I answer. "Yes, I eat properly."

"Do you get enough rest?" she asks.

My friends and I talk, but about money, work, relationships, children. No one else asks me these basic questions. Am I surviving? No one dares get so deep, so primal.

In the beginning, the mother is *the* everything, the arms and heart and breath of her daughter. The mother is the leader, the model. She takes a step and her daughter follows. But gradually, the child pushes away from her mother. Like a swimmer, kicking off from the side of the pool, the child moves herself into deeper water.

I know that moment, that standing alone at the edge of the pool, watching my daughter swim faster and farther. It is a moment of hallelujah-success and heartbreak-loneliness. To be a good mother means to lose your child to the world.

My mother's child has returned. I am old enough to allow her to renew our original bond, my original role in life. I am old enough that I truly treasure having a mother.

This is a book about learning from my mother through the stages of her Alzheimer's. It is the story of our family's journey with my mother and her Alzheimer's disease, a story of *Love in the Land of Dementia*.

My story starts with a handwritten letter, circa 1948. In careful, blocky printing, Paul Barnett, a man whose wife divorced him while he was stationed in England during World War II, writes to his best friend Max that he is ready to settle down with a nice Jewish girl. Paul wants a woman who shares his values, who wants children, and who can make wonderful brownies.

Max shows the letter to his wife, Bel, who shows the letter to her best friend Fran.

"You remember Paul, don't you?" Bel asks Fran. "You met him in England, at the dance. He was married at the time, but his wife left him."

Fran shakes her head. She vaguely remembers meeting a serious-looking, uniformed man named Paul, but she can't bring his face to mind.

"He's a nice guy," Bel says. "And he wants to meet someone. I'm writing him back. You should put a P.S. on my letter."

Fran lowers her head and turns down the corner of page 242 in her political science text. Although she is already a registered nurse (RN), she does not have a college degree and she's studying at the University of Colorado in Boulder. Her first husband died years earlier, and she became an army nurse to get away from her grief.

Since she has been out of the service, Fran has been wondering if she'll meet someone again, someone to raise a family with. Bel dashes off a breezy letter to Paul, and Fran adds this scintillating P.S.—"Hi, Paul. Remember me from England? Frances."

Those scrawled words began a correspondence that resulted in the marriage of my parents, Paul Barnett and Frances Shinbaum, on October 10, 1948.

When my father passed away we found a stack of his letters to Mom neatly tucked into his pajama drawer. They were waiting for us.

My father's letters showed me the other side of my parents' love story, the true story my mother did not like to admit to.

Years before, when I had asked my mother about her early relationship with Dad, she told me, "We had similar values. We both wanted to raise a family. We weren't in love when we married, but we learned to love each other."

I had never questioned Dad about the early years—in our family, relationship conversations were Mom's territory. That changed only when Mom was deep into Alzheimer's. During that period, when I asked Dad, "How long did it take you to fall in love with Mom after you married?" he looked at me quizzically, then answered, "Not very long at all."

I imagine my father and mother saving each other's letters. The letters moved with them from Manchester, New Hampshire, to Gulfport, Mississippi, to Wynne, Arkansas, to Memphis, Tennessee. In Memphis, the letters settled: Mom's in her underwear drawer, Dad's in his pajama drawer. Perhaps Mom's were tied with a ribbon; Dad's were held together by a rubber band. When my mother had her first bout with heart problems, she would have considered what to do with those letters. She would have thought about dying young, as her mother did, and about my brother and me, ages ten and eight at the time, someday reading all those letters. She would have called my dad aside, and together, late one night, they would have read through everything, laughing and leaning against each other. Then Mom would have carefully torn up most of her letters and the letters of Dad's that were too racy (I'm sure they argued over the raciness quotient) and my father would have put the uncensored letters back in his pajama drawer.

Dad's letters show the real story—from the second letter, he was already deeply, passionately in love with Mom. During the years of Mom's Alzheimer's, I was privileged to experience the truth and depth of my father's love.

I.
Confusion:
THE EARLY STAGES,
1997–1998

Leaving the Purse Behind

"I want a divorce." The long-distance call from my father comes at four o'clock on a Sunday afternoon. "Your mother and I can no longer live together, and I'm going to get a divorce."

These are the reasons my father wants a divorce: My mother, Fran, is changing. She is snippy, forgetful, and downright irritating. She misplaces everything so many times a day that it's like rounding up the toys of a two-year-old. Dad plans a nice day for them—swimming, lunch at a favorite restaurant, then a movie—the kind of day they both love. She sabotages it. First, she can't find her swimsuit, which for forty years has lived in the top right drawer of her dresser. Then her swim cap is gone. She packs her shampoo and conditioner, and when she gets into the car they have somehow escaped from her bag. She can't leave the house without taking a drink of water. Then, by the time she reaches the front door, she needs another drink of water.

"Take the glass with you," my father says, his voice reaching a loud and angry edge.

"Don't talk to me like that," my mother says.

The timing of the perfect day is already off. They leave the house a half-hour later than planned, which means the indoor pool will already be crowded and my dad's lap swimming will be chaotic.

He walks my mother to the women's dressing room and goes right to the pool. He knows after he swims for ten minutes, he'll feel better. After she swims for a few minutes, Mom will feel better, too. Then, they'll laugh about whatever was going on back home. They'll be in the water together, like they've been so many times over the years; my father with his stroke still strong and my mother moving with rubber-ducky speed, one hand over the other, a slow-motion ballet punctuated with a single emphatic kick and a breath.

So my father swims laps, moving back into calm and steadiness. After a while, he looks up to wave at my mother and notices she is not yet at the pool. He looks at the clock and sees that ten minutes have passed. He is not yet worried, since she is so slow these days, so lost in some maze of her own peculiar design. As he swims, he remembers being in the ocean with her and with my brother and me as children, and he smiles underwater. Even in the rambunctious ocean waves, his wife maintains her slow, steady crawl stroke, and that is just one of the things he enjoys about her. He's now ready to swim over to her underwater, surprising her with a kiss on her knees, but she's still not in the pool.

He climbs up the ladder, goes to the lifeguard, and says, "My wife has not come out of the dressing room yet and I'm worried about her."

The lifeguard wears a whistle, a University of Memphis T-shirt, and boxy blue swim trunks. He runs his hand through his blond buzz cut, walks over to the phone on the wall, and calls the lady at the towel desk.

"She's going to check," he tells Dad.

Dad's edginess takes over his throat and his chest. He waits by the door of the women's dressing room, imagining Fran fallen onto the floor, cut and bleeding. He is so sorry he snapped at her this morning, and vows that if she's all right he'll be more patient. He closes his eyes, ignores the chill he feels, and prays that she is all right. Just then the towel lady leads Mom out. Mom is wearing her usual yellow flip-flops, carrying her usual plastic bag with the towel and shampoo inside it, wearing her fuchsia-and-black swimsuit that she still looks good in.

"I couldn't find the door to the pool," she tells Dad, smiling and shaking her head. "I was just wandering around that dressing room, and finally this nice lady came and led me right to the door."

Dad gives her a wet hug. He tries to smile. He pretends his tears are drops of pool water.

Mom gets into the pool, leaving her flip-flops right beside the ladder as always, and swims her leisurely, loopy stroke, as always.

"Do you need help finding your way around the dressing room?" Dad asks as they are getting out.

"I think I'm fine now," she says. "I'm sorry if I worried you; I was feeling pretty darn frustrated myself."

Dad kisses her cheek and they go to their separate dressing rooms. Fifteen minutes after Dad has come out, Mom emerges, like always. She's looking fresh and happy. They hold hands walking to the car.

"Let's go to the Pancake House," Dad says. He knows how Mom loves to eat pancakes in the middle of the day.

She doesn't say anything.

"Fran, what about the Pancake House?" He raises his voice, but just a little, so she won't accuse him of shouting at her.

She looks out the car window, then glances at him and smiles.

"Did you hear what I said?" he asks, now making his voice even louder.

"No, dear. What did you say?"

Dad notices that Mom is not wearing her hearing aids. He tries to remember if she was wearing them when they left the house; he's pretty sure she was. Now he struggles to recall if she was wearing them when she went into the pool; he hopes she was not.

"Where are your hearing aids?" he asks, now knowing exactly how loudly to speak so she can hear him.

She touches her ears. "I must have left them in the dressing room. I had a feeling I was forgetting something but I couldn't think what."

Dad feels a wave of exhaustion, anger, and despair rise through him, and he bites his mouth shut against it.

"Wait here," he says, and he rushes back to the towel lady to tell her his problem. The towel lady goes into the women's dressing room; a few minutes later she emerges with the hearing aid container.

"On one of the sinks," she reports. "Looks like the hearing aids are both here." She hands the container to my father. "Take care of yourself," she says softly. "Take care of her, too."

The softness of her voice goes right into the place Dad has been avoiding all morning, the sad, lost part that wants to wail and rant over this unexpected turn in life. He wants to fall apart and have everything be all right when he gets it all together again. But for now, he races back to the car, praying she is sitting exactly where he left her.

She is.

"Thank you, honey," she says as she inserts her hearing aids. "That was so nice of you."

There is still that sweetness, that wonderful connection they have always shared. But the smoothness of their life together is gone. At any moment, a hesitation, stubbornness, a lost item, a repeated question, what was it you said, for the fourth and fifth time, jars my father into anxiety and confusion. The losing and finding rituals make it almost impossible to leave the house without wanting to shout.

My brother and I try to help.

A counselor, we suggest. A neurologist. A gerontologist. We search for therapies that will catapult Mom from this haze of forgetfulness. Natural hormones, we suggest. Vitamin C, music therapy, drinking lots of water, getting enough sunshine, ginkgo, etc. Every week we call Dad and gently offer ideas.

Meanwhile, Dad and Mom are enmeshed with the neurologist, the gerontologist, the social worker, and the psychologist, who all talk about the possibility of Alzheimer's disease. Dad is conducting his own research. One of his friends' daughters conquered depression with a copper bracelet; isn't this forgetfulness of Mom's a form of depression? He reads about magnets and designs a hat with a brim of magnets that Mom can wear around the house. He keeps Mom moving, walking, swimming, and takes her out to eat, to movies, to jazz clubs. Movement is a key to good mental health, and he figures he'll move her right through whatever this is. But she takes a few steps and stops, stuck.

"She's testing me," Dad says when he calls. "I can't take it much longer."

"Your father seems so impatient," Mom says, her voice small and tentative. "He yells at me all the time."

"Are you putting in your hearing aids, Mom?" I ask. "Maybe he's talking loudly so you can hear."

"What, dear?" Mom asks. "What did you say?"

I picture the hearing aids, forgotten in some drawer or on some sink counter, or in some cabinet.

My mother gets off the airplane looking like she's landed on a foreign planet and has no idea what the atmosphere is like. A flight attendant escorts her, and Mom clings to her arm. Then Mom finally notices me and smiles.

"Oh, it's you," she says, hugging me fiercely. "I wondered what all this was about."

I too have wondered what all this is about, and I am getting a chance to see and experience my father's current life. My mother is visiting me for a week so my father can have a break.

When my mother was safely in Memphis, I had wondered if my father was simply impatient, expecting too much from her. I wondered if they were in some sort of quarrel. But now, after only two days of living with Mom, I am already feeling the frazzle and frustration my dad described. Only two days.

Now that my mother is here and I am the one repeating answers and unearthing lost objects—the misplaced glasses, the lost purse, the forgotten hearing aids; the endless barrage of questions, what time are we leaving, what time did you say we are leaving, when should I be ready, are we going someplace?—I understand how pale and weak the words of advice I have been giving my father were.

"I can't leave the house without my purse," my mother now says, her voice stern. My father had warned me about the purse, about how it could walk, run, hide, burrow behind books, under beds, under rugs, and behind ancient, crusted bottles of talcum powder in the bathroom closet that nobody ever uses anymore. I search, and the purse eludes me.

"I can't leave without my purse," Mom says when I urge her again to get ready.

I have given us a full half-hour of extra time, time to go again to the bathroom, get the extra sips of water, and find the already lost and misplaced items. I realize thirty minutes is not nearly long enough.

I look again in the secret places the purse has already discovered in my house—under the pillow, in the kitchen cabinet, under the bed, in the bathtub. Not there.

"Mom, what do you need from your purse?" I ask as the moments march by and our lateness looms large.

"My money, my driver's license, my tissues," she explains.

"Tell you what. I have money and I'm treating today. I'm driving, and I'll put extra tissues in my pockets. Let's go ahead just this once without the purse. You'll have everything you need."

Mom stops and thinks about this. "All right," she says. "It's just an old purse, after all."

One moment the purse is a vital, pulsing necessity, a principle worth fighting over, and a moment later it's just another material object. I smile at my mother's unintended wisdom, the beauty of the slipped memory, the mystical mind, that lapse of synapse that allows her to doggedly hang on and then laughingly let go.

"Where are we going?" Mom asks for the fourth time as I start the car.

It's a simple question—one I really don't know how to answer.

Reading Lessons

"What does that say?" Dad asks, from the backseat, as we pass a billboard with a bright picture of a donut.

"Dunk in and delight," my mother reads.

Several months have passed, and I'm visiting my parents in Memphis. I am driving them to their new favorite Chinese restaurant. Their old favorite restaurant is under new management and, according to my father, the crab Rangoon, the wonton soup, and the fried rice have all suffered from the change.

As I pull into the parking lot, my father asks Mom, "What did that billboard say?"

"What billboard, dear?" Mom asks, turning slightly in her seat to give Dad a sweet smile.

Inside the restaurant, the proprietress greets Dad with a big grin and a warm handshake.

"Mr. Barnett. Mrs. Barnett. And this must be your daughter. We love having your parents come eat with us. We wish they'd eat with us every night."

A girl of about four years old runs between the tables and clamps her arms around her mother's leg. The girl tilts her head to smile at my father.

"Hello," my father says. "Do you want a piece of bubble gum?"

Her short black hair swings as she nods yes.

Dad reaches into his pocket for a piece of gum, then takes Mom's arm and leads her to a table. I sit opposite them.

"Who was that lovely child?" my mother asks when we are settled with menus and water. "What a beautiful little girl."

"That's Mellie, the owner's daughter. You remember her. She brought you a fortune cookie when we were here last week. She read you a chapter out of her storybook."

Mom smiles, a conciliatory smile that is becoming her standard. The smile is her shield, her plea, her apologia for all she might have accidentally forgotten.

"What do I like here?" Mom asks, looking at the large menu.

"Wonton soup, sweet and sour chicken, pork fried rice," Dad tells her. These are the same dishes Mom has been ordering since I was a child.

As we eat our dinner, my father returns to their dilemma, the dilemma we have been discussing over the phone.

"Your mother just doesn't seem to be concentrating anymore. Like that billboard: She sees the billboard, she reads the words, and a minute later she can't remember them."

"It's true," Mom says, shaking her head ruefully. "I can't remember. There's nothing I can do about it, so I don't get too upset. Paul, I wish you wouldn't get so upset."

"I just want you to concentrate more," he says, taking a spoonful of soup.

My father is the third-born child of two Russian peasant immigrants. His father ran away to Barnet, England, fought in the Boer War, and later worked on the Panama Canal. He thrived on overcoming adversity and challenges. My father also understands adversity and challenge. He will conquer any villain to save the woman he loves. Meanwhile, the woman he loves, the daughter of Polish and Hungarian immigrants, stares at the two slim sticks resting beside her plate—chopsticks that she has always enjoyed eating rice with—shakes her head, and picks up a fork.

That same weekend, I take Mom to the seventy-fifth birthday party of her dear friend Elaine. No men are invited, so I am going as her chauffeur and her spokeswoman.

I always like it when my father hands me the car keys. Hearing the keys jingle out of his pockets and into my waiting palm reminds me of those long-ago days when borrowing the car was a major coup. Borrowing the car meant I had our family's only mode of transportation in my sweating teenage hands. Now my hands are sweating because I have not been alone with Mom since she spent that week with me.

As Mom and I drive through the neighborhoods, she suddenly asks, "How's work going?"

Even though she has asked me this question many times already during my short visit, I answer again. I pretend this is a creativity exercise. My job is to answer the same question in a new and different way each time.

"How are the kids?" she asks when I pause. I see how artfully she steers me into monologue, punctuated by her simple questions.

As I park the car, Mom says, "Where are we going?"

"We're at Elaine's. It's her seventy-fifth birthday party."

"Oh yes. Of course. Are you coming with me?"

"I'll be right beside you," I say, patting her hand.

"That's good."

Elaine's living room is teeming with women. Mom's face tightens as someone rushes over to greet her. "So good to see you, Fran," Mom's old friend Poppy says, giving Mom a hug. "And you, Debbie, you look great," she says to me.

Elaine comes up to greet us.

"How are you, Fran?" Elaine says in a low, concerned voice.

"I don't know," Mom answers, her voice so small and scared that I feel a well of sadness. I remember walking into the house when I was a girl and finding Mom lying unconscious on the hallway floor. I remember the helpless fear that shook me, even while I tried to revive her and then called our neighbor and the ambulance. During the ambulance ride, Mom rallied. She'd had an attack of tachycardia—rapid heartbeat—and had fainted. And now, even though she's standing upright, looking beautiful in her turquoise dress and carefully applied red lipstick, I feel her helplessness and I am afraid.

I guide her to the food table, and we each select tiny sandwiches, curly carrots, saltine crackers with chopped liver, and sweet pink cakes. Then I take her into the den, where we sit together on the sofa, near old friends from the days when Mom taught Sunday school.

"So, Debbie, how are you? How are your kids? What are you doing?" some of the women ask me.

Beside me, I feel my mother relaxing as the conversation points to me.

"Fran, what are you reading these days? Did you finish that Isaac Singer book I told you about?" Gerda asks.

Anxiety pinches Mom's face.

"Mom hasn't had much time to read," I tell Gerda. I wonder if Gerda doesn't know or just doesn't want to admit that her friend of forty years is changing. I wonder if seeing those changes frightens her as much as it sometimes terrifies me.

The conversation swirls around us as more of Mom's friends gather in the den. I sit beside my mother and field her questions, as if she were a politician with something to hide. As I talk, Mom again starts to relax, smile, and laugh. She is enjoying being around her friends without having to come up with answers. She is liberated from her forgetfulness and having fun just listening, being here, and eating the sweet pink cakes.

When it's time to go, Mom and I each hug Elaine good-bye.

"You take care of her," Elaine says.

"I will," I say.

"Thank you," Mom says as we walk to the car. She takes my hand, and I feel a sweet sadness at this surprising and vulnerable gesture.

I imagine, or rather I try to imagine, what Mom must be going through, wanting to connect, to talk to people, and all the while having a mind as blank and frozen as a winter pond. I imagine the anxiety that must come with each social encounter: Are they going to ask a direct question? Are they going to refer to something that happened earlier? Do they expect certain questions back?

"This must be so hard," I say as I drive home.

"It is," Mom says. "But there's nothing to do but let it go and laugh it off. Otherwise, I go crazy."

Back home, my father is in his recliner, reading the newspaper. We tell him about the party and I describe all the different people we saw. He looks pleased.

My mother gets herself a cup of coffee and settles near him on the sofa, with a book. I sit on the other end of the sofa, with my book.

We are all in our places. The setting is familiar and comforting, as long as I try not to notice that Mom is holding the book open, upside down on her lap, staring ahead as though all she can read is the future.

Let It Be

For the first time, my mother cannot really help prepare our seder meal. She wanders around the kitchen, pausing at the counter, the stove, the table as if to collect something lost.

"What was I doing?" she asks.

"Setting the table," I say.

"How many people are coming?"

"Ten," I say, spilling the spoonful of oil in my irritation. An old football cheer floats into my mind: "First and ten, do it again. Do it again." And again. Mom has already asked me these questions several times in the last ten minutes.

When Mom and Dad drove up two days ago, Dad's face was tight, and he went straight to the guest room to take a nap.

"Sometimes I wish I were hard of hearing," he told me later that evening.

Mom's speech is like an old record player with a needle that refuses to leave its groove. The simple anchors of life—the who, what, where, and when of things—often elude her.

"Did you remember the macaroons for dessert?" she asks, fork in hand.

"Yes," I say, again. I crack an egg and have to scoop shell out of the bowl.

I stir the matzo mixture and take a breath. I have trained myself to be brisk and efficient, but now, around my mother, I need to be slow and soft.

"How many people are coming?" she asks.

"Ten," I say, impatience pinching my throat. "Let's take a break and go for a walk."

I wipe my hands and look for the house keys. They are not on their usual hook in the cabinet. They are not in my purse, or lolling on the kitchen table. I feel a brief flutter of shame over the impatience I felt just this morning, when Mom misplaced her glasses case for the second time. Then I feel a stab of fear: Am I, too, losing my mind?

"Have you seen my keys?" I ask my daughter, who comes breezing through, searching for chocolate to inspire her midterm studying.

She stops, Hershey's bar in hand. "They're right in front of you, Mom," she says, pointing to a huddled mass of metal on the counter corner. I pocket the keys and double-check to make sure I have turned off the stove.

Outside, the redbuds are flowering, the dogwoods skirting newly green lawns. My mother and I walk past a closed-down lemonade stand—three broken lawn chairs set out on the curb and a blond, floppy-haired girl skipping over a pink jump rope.

"It was hard when my mother died. My father just disappeared, took off walking," Mom says. "He was a good man, though."

I nod. I remember as much about my mother's childhood as I do my own. The story of her mother's death is one in a series of memories Mom has told me all my life.

We pass a woman with a sleeping baby in a stroller, and Mom smiles.

"Did you get the macaroons?"

"Yes, I did, Mom."

"Did I already ask you that?"

"Yes."

"Your father gets mad at me sometimes," she says. "He thinks I'm forgetting on purpose."

"What's it like to not remember?" I ask.

An eager black spaniel rushes up to us.

"I start a thought," Mom says, bending to pet the dog, "and the end disappears. If I try too hard to catch it, that makes it worse. So I let go, and eventually I get the answer. Of course, by that time, something else is going on." Mom smiles and shakes her head. Her hair is silvery and curly, her hands like fine dried flowers, her stride crisp and full.

All weekend I have watched her happily listen to the conversations around her, passionately asking a question, then moments later, equally passionately, asking the same question. I have listened to her stories, which have the comforting familiarity of a well-worn quilt. These stories, which were sprinkled throughout my growing-up years, are now the major part of our conversations.

That evening, we celebrate Passover with a seder service. As the service progresses, my father tells our guests about *Dayenu,* a Hebrew word that means "Even that would have been enough."

"It sounds like *Die-aa-nu,*" he says. "You repeat it after each of the sentences I'm going to read. It's a way of expressing gratitude."

My mother fiddles with the prayer book and asks for the third time, "Is it time for Elijah?"

"Not yet," my father says, his voice tense. Then he calms and begins the Dayenu litany:

"If God had divided the sea without leading us onto dry land . . ."

"Dayenu," we all intone.

"If God had taken care of us in the desert for forty years without feeding us manna . . ."

"Dayenu."

"If God had fed us manna without . . ."

And so we follow the journey of our ancestors, promising we will be satisfied. With whatever we get.

As I repeat my gratitude and pledge my satisfaction with life as it is, I think of my mother. I miss her remembering all the details of my life. I miss her knowing where the silverware drawer is. I miss telling her something I'm proud of and having her remember it. And yet, she is the living symbol of Dayenu, graciously accepting her failing mind and making the best of it.

"And now, it's time to eat," my father says.

My mother reaches over and pats my wrist. I see the patina of softness that burnishes her, the loving core that goes far beyond mundane daily detail. I see the woman who has loved me even during the years I wandered through a difficult wilderness.

As we sip our sweet wine and break off a piece of unleavened bread, I create my own litany:

If my mother gets pleasure out of life . . .

Dayenu.

If she remembers who I am . . .

Dayenu.

"This is a lovely seder," she says. "You did a beautiful job of putting all this together."

I press her hand, look into her smiling face, and say, "Dayenu."

The Stroke

I pick up the phone and hear my father cry for the first time in my life.

"I had a stroke," he says, sobbing. "I'm in the hospital."

For a moment, I can't speak. I am petrified by the sound of my father's small and broken voice.

"Are you all right?" I ask.

"Yes, I am. My speech is a little slurred, that's all. The therapist says I will recover."

"Where is Mom?"

"She's sitting right here. The nurses are helping me look after her."

"I'll be there as soon as I find a flight," I say, my hands trembling.

"Thank you, darling," my father says, his words swallowed into tears.

I hang up the phone and just stand there. My father usually says, "Don't bother. I'm all right. I can handle it," no matter what he's going through. I am immobilized by his desire for my help. I cannot pick up the phone book and find the airline number. I cannot wait on hold while cheerful music plays and a perky voice promises that my call is important.

I am near tears as I call my daughter. She quickly takes charge, gets me a flight, and then comes over to help me pack. She drives me to the airport. Within two hours, I am sitting numbly on a plane to Memphis.

My father is entangled in a network of tubes. My mother sits nearby, her hands clenched and her eyes blank and lost.

I hug her, then lean down to gently hug Dad. His eyes tear up.

"I can't seem to stop crying," he says. "That stroke must have burst a tear duct."

"You look great," I say, relieved at how strong his speech is, how normal his face. "What happened?"

He and Mom were almost finished with their usual early-evening stroll. Suddenly, he felt a flash of severe discomfort and numbness in his leg. Next thing, he was lying on the ground, with my mother kneeling over him, shaking him. She helped him up and helped him home. But his leg didn't seem to work.

"I need to go to the hospital," he told my mother. "Do you think you can drive me?"

"What?" I interrupt his story. "Mom drove you to the hospital? Mom isn't supposed to drive. How come you didn't call an ambulance?" My voice is rising.

"I didn't want to bother. Your mother said she could do it and I knew she would."

I twist my hands as Dad describes the harrowing drive through rush-hour traffic. As her Alzheimer's has advanced, Mom has developed a habit of sitting still at stop signs and smiling sweetly when the people behind her honk. Occasionally, she totally ignores a stop sign. She had not driven in months. Dad struggled to remain alert and coherent as he reintroduced Mom to the accelerator and brake and prayed she didn't get confused. He had to tell Mom when to turn, when to stop, and how fast to go.

"My words were coming out funny," he says, "and sometimes they got stuck. But we made it."

I put my hands over my eyes and shudder as I imagine Mom driving my father to this hospital. She cannot always remember how to turn on the tap water or put the toothpaste on her brush. Yet somehow she maneuvered the car and got her husband here safely. I am grateful for this miracle.

"Where's the car?" I ask.

"Somewhere in the hospital parking lot. Your mother didn't want to leave me. But now that you're here, I figure you can take her home for a rest."

I talk to the doctor, the speech therapist, and the social worker. They assure me Dad will be fine. He will fully recover his speech. He hasn't lost any movement or mobility. He was very lucky, they tell me.

Mom and I go out to the visitor's parking lot and start searching for the car. Mom holds my hand. It is growing dark when we finally find it. We stop by the grocery store on the way home and I ask Mom if she needs anything.

"Ice cream and milk," she says.

I buy fruit, milk, and ingredients for dinner, and Mom selects two gallons of chocolate ice cream.

Back home, I open the freezer door and see six gallons of the same chocolate ice cream and one sack of peas. I shove in the cartons and make us dinner. The house seems quiet with just the two of us. Mom walks restlessly around the den, picking up a stack of mail and carrying it into the dining room, then to the living room. Finally, she carries a few of the letters back into the den and sets them on another stack.

Normally, my parents have a tidy home. Mom likes order. But I now see these towers of mail are scattered around the house. Mom barely eats her meal. She goes to the freezer and gets some ice cream. She has always loved sweets, and this consistency comforts me. I'd like to go back to the hospital and check on Dad, yet I see how tired she is. I don't want to leave her alone.

I call Dad.

"Don't worry about coming back here tonight," he says. "I'm fine. I am thinking, though . . ." He pauses. "I am thinking maybe it's time we move up to Kansas City, to be closer to you."

"Good idea," I say.

For years, Dad has been toying with the idea of moving to Kansas City. For years, Dad has explored apartments, houses, and retirement communities in the area. Now, he's finally ready.

I look at my watch and try to calculate the time in Tokyo, where my brother now lives. I want to talk to him, to tell him about Dad, and about Dad being ready to move to Kansas City. But I don't want to scare Daniel with a dramatic late-night call. I decide to wait until it's his early morning.

Mom's in the den, still fiddling with the mail. She rearranges the letters with great seriousness. I sit on the old sofa. We built this den when I was ten years old and all our neighbors were also adding onto their houses. I remember how glamorous it felt to have such a room, with its hardwood floors and fireplace.

The familiar photo albums still cover the coffee table. I know what's in each one: pictures of my childhood and our family travels, pictures of my children, pictures of my brother's children and of my parents' travels. I know the story of each knickknack on the mantle. I have leafed through every book in the built-in bookcase and examined every photograph, painting, and plaque on the wall. I can't imagine packing up everything in this house. Yet I can't imagine my parents continuing to stay here.

Mom goes off to her room and I settle into my old bedroom, keeping the door open in case Mom needs anything. I take the portable phone from the kitchen and call Ron, my life partner. Just hearing his voice soothes me, and I spill out the story of Mom driving Dad to the emergency room.

"Your father is so independent," Ron says. "He's also very lucky."

Ron is fueled by that same sort of independence, determination, and persistence. After he has described his day and I feel anchored once again, I call my brother. I have rehearsed my opening words.

"Dad's all right. But he had a stroke."

"What!" Daniel is startled.

I tell him the whole story and he listens intently.

"Do you need me to come?" he asks.

"I think we'll need you more when they get ready to move," I say, although the thought of my brother being here with me in our growing-up house holds a promise of tremendous comfort.

"I can't believe this," he says, and I hear how hard it is for him to be so far away.

I tell him about Mom's freezer full of chocolate ice cream, and he laughs.

After the conversation, I lie down. My old dresser is now filled with Mom's art supplies, but some of my books are still on the bookshelf along with a fragile clay figure of a woman that an admirer once sent me.

A couple of hours into sleep, I hear Mom walking around in the den and the kitchen. I get up to see if she's okay, squinting against the lights.

"I can't find your father," she says, a carton of ice cream on the counter and a bowl and spoon on the stove.

"He's in the hospital," I remind her.

"Oh yes. I forgot. Is he okay?"

"Yes, he is. We'll go visit him tomorrow."

Mom looks so vulnerable and scared, standing in her kitchen wearing the forest-green silk robe Dad got her two anniversaries ago over her ancient pink sateen pajamas. I reach out my arms and we hug. I feel a sudden warmth and realize she has turned on the stove. The burner is glowing red; the teakettle waits quietly in the sink.

"Did you want some coffee?" I ask.

"Yes," she says.

"And some ice cream?"

"That would be lovely."

"I'll get us both some," I say.

I serve Mom and sit beside her on the sofa. I take a spoonful of ice cream and realize my life is changing. I am going to lose my childhood home and I am also going to lose my familiar relationship with my parents. Mom pats my leg. I lean my head against her shoulder. She leans her head on mine.

"This is good," she says.

For a moment, I feel peaceful and safe. Then Mom stands and picks up a stack of junk mail. She looks carefully at each letter, and then carries the stack into the bathroom.

Our Last Summer Vacation

I hold my mother's hand as we walk down the flagstone path to the pool.

"Where is . . .?" she asks again, her voice filled with the ache of the missing word.

I squeeze her hand. "Dad is resting this morning," I tell her. "He'll meet us at the pool later."

She nods and grips my hand.

"She doesn't want me out of her sight," my dad had told me over the phone as we planned this family reunion. For years, our family has met annually at this vintage resort in Hot Springs, Arkansas. My parents brought my brother and me here when we were young, and Dad rediscovered the place some years ago—a venue with enough activities for the kids and enough relaxation for the adults. Dad has recovered beautifully from his stroke and did not want to give up our traditional family gathering. But we all realize this may be our last time here.

A dragonfly flits by and a cardinal perches on a nearby branch. Mom looks at the brilliant red bird and smiles. Then her face becomes a map of anxiety.

I open the gate to the pool and usher Mom to a chair beside an umbrella-topped table.

"Where is . . .?" she asks.

"He'll be here soon," I say, sitting down beside her, trying not to show my own nervousness.

Last night, I had told my father, "I'll spend the day with Mom, and you take a break."

"I don't know if I can take a break," he told me, tears gathering in his eyes.

"Try. I'll take care of Mom."

This morning, when Mom woke up, Dad walked her over to my room. I brought her inside, talking animatedly to her as Dad walked away.

Only seconds after he left, Mom looked around as though she'd misplaced something valuable. Her hands shivered and her face tightened.

"Where is . . .?" she asked.

"He's resting this morning," I said, leading her to the little kitchenette table. "You and I get to hang out together this morning."

"Yes, that's nice," she said as I prepared her breakfast of coffee, milk, juice, toast, and a sliced orange. But I could feel her worry, her unease. I feel my own worry: Will I be able to keep her calm and content for the next several hours?

The pool is empty this morning. I wonder if the water might be too cold for Mom, yet I know Dad has been bringing her swimming every morning. Perhaps my nephew Jake will show up, bold and boyish and full of energy. Or his older brother, Zachary—this summer sporting bright blond spiked hair. Zachary is not afraid of his grandmother's forgetfulness. Perhaps Helen, their older sister, might stroll through, her swollen belly golden and glowing with six months' worth of child.

"Nana, put your hand right here, on my stomach. See if you can feel the baby kicking," Helen might say.

My daughter Hilee, full of warmth and compassion, might wander out to the pool to see if her grandmother needs a drink of ice water or a slice of orange. Or Sarah, my younger daughter who just graduated from college, might stroll up, trying to understand what is happening and what it means to everyone.

Meanwhile, I sit with my mother and point out the various trees, flowers, and birds around us. I feel like I am taking care of someone else's child, a child who at any minute might burst into wails and want her real mother NOW. I'd like my real mother now. My real mother would stop clutching the towel and get into the pool with me. We would swim together, and then my real mother would get out, towel off, and go take a shower. We would meet again to talk and read.

My brother Daniel is the first one to arrive at the pool. He's carrying a towel, a bottle of water, and a thick suspense novel.

"Hi, Mom," he says. She smiles at him.

"Where's Dad?" he asks, quietly.

"He's taking part of the day off," I tell him.

"Good, that's good," Daniel says.

Neither one of us knows exactly what to do, what to say, how to act around Mom.

I remember the summer, ten years ago, when Daniel and I, each in the throes of postdivorce therapy, decided we would ask our parents why they hadn't appreciated us more when we were growing up. Both of us had felt we were never "enough" for our parents, and both of us were now working hard to believe in our own worth.

Daniel would talk to Dad, as his therapist had encouraged him to, and I would talk to Mom, as my therapist had encouraged me to. Daniel and I had several nervous conversations, deciding just when to have these talks and what to say: We did not want to be confrontational (or so we believed)—we just wanted to understand more. Finally, the last afternoon of our stay, Daniel went for a walk with Dad. Mom and I sat near the dock, at a weathered picnic table. After a long silence, I took a breath and said, "How come you didn't ever praise me or act like I was smart or special when I was growing up? I think I was a pretty good kid. But I never felt that you really loved or approved of me." My heart thudded as I said these words.

Mom looked at the lake, then lowered her head. "I did love you but I didn't want you to feel loved," she answered matter-of-factly. "I always felt so special when I was a child. Then my mother died and suddenly I didn't feel special anymore. I didn't want you to have to go through that. I figured if you didn't feel so loved, you wouldn't ever have to suffer such a loss."

The picnic table's splintery wood was warm against my palms as I let my mother's words fall into me. She had been trying to keep me safe from heartbreak. This had been her parenting plan, born of her own traumatic and motherless adolescence. I felt a deep sadness and sense of loss at the poignancy of such thinking.

"Maybe I made a mistake," Mom said, looking at me with concern.

"No, it's okay, Mom," I answered, feeling empty rather than hurt. "I just wanted to understand."

When my brother and I conferred later that evening, we were both somber as we shared our stories. Dad hadn't remembered any of the incidents that had troubled my brother.

"I'm sorry if I hurt your feelings," Dad said. And then he added, "That was a long time ago."

Now those conversations seem like ages ago.

"Where is . . .?" Mom asks, her hands knotting together.

"He's resting," I say. "Let's go swimming."

Now that my brother is here, I feel comfortable taking Mom into the pool. I feel confident that the two of us can get her in and out, if somehow she forgets how to navigate the steps.

I take Mom's hand. We go down the large concrete steps, built for toddlers, and wade into the shallow water.

"Nice," Mom says. "We used to go into the hot springs in Iceland, during the war. We would be skiing from one place to the next, and there would be a hot spring, just steaming by the side of the road. We'd get in, get warmed up, then continue on our way."

I smile. Now we are in safe territory—remembrances of her army nurse days during World War II. Now we are in a talking terrain where I can ask questions and invite stories, and Mom can easily roll them out.

We walk around in the shallow water, and Mom tells wartime stories. My brother sits by the side of the pool and reads. By the time my father shows up, we are connected and calm.

Mom waves and smiles. "Paul, over here, Paul." Underneath her smile I hear the relief in her voice.

My father gets into the pool and warmly greets Mom.

"I'm going to swim," he tells her.

"Okay, dear."

"Is she all right?" he asks me, though he has been away from her for only two hours.

"She's fine. She asked about you and I told her you were resting."

"And she was okay?"

"Yes, she was okay."

Dad nods and begins his lap swimming.

That afternoon, I fix Mom lunch and we sit together in my room. It's blazing hot outside, and Mom does not like such heat. Dad, Daniel, and the children have gone into town to go bowling and play pool. Mom and I are having a "girls'" afternoon.

After eating, I take out the drawing supplies I have brought. We sit at the table and I hand Mom a pad of paper and spread crayons, markers, and pencils in front of her.

"Let's sketch together," I suggest. Mom is an accomplished artist whose paintings enliven my parents' home. But in the last several years, she has not been near her art.

I begin a primitive drawing, letting intuition guide my hand. I am engrossed in following my own lines of thought, adding splashes of color without design or forethought. I look over at Mom—she is moving a yellow crayon rhythmically back and forth so that the page is a swarm of blinding yellow.

"I really need to go home now," Mom says. "The light is hurting my eyes."

I pull down the shades and dim the lights.

"Let's just sit together," I say. "I'll make us some coffee and we'll talk."

"All right," she says.

I make us coffee, put some cookies on a plate, and settle myself next to Mom. I feel her anxiety, her desire to be someplace else—with Dad, I imagine.

She reaches for a cookie.

"I'm sorry I can't remember your name," Mom says. "I can't remember any of their names."

I feel like I have been punched in the stomach. My mother cannot remember my name. My mother, the creator of me and bestower of my name, no longer knows me. My throat grows tight with the immensity of this thought. Part of me wants to bolt out of the room, to get away from this woman and the words she just said. Another part of me wants to grab her by the shoulders, look her in the eyes, and repeat my name over and over until it is impossible for her to forget it. But I realize that is what my father has been trying to do for months, with no success.

"I'm sorry," Mom says, her face solemn.

"It's okay, Mom." Tears well up as I put my arm around her. "We all understand." But I don't understand. Can't she just remember these three names: Debbie, Dan, and Paul? Three words, thirteen letters; can't she at least remember that?

"It's sad," she says, clenching her hands.

"It is sad," I agree, touching her shoulder. "And I know it's hard on you."

"Yes," she says. "You can't imagine."

I have imagined, waking Ron up in the middle of too many black nights, what it might be like. I have tasted that jolt of fear and helplessness, when I too have forgotten simple things. But I know that I truly cannot imagine the minute-to-minute stress and confusion Mom is going through.

We sit there in the dark, my mother and I, sipping coffee, eating cookies, and letting the world rush past without us. We sit quietly, a mother who didn't want her daughter to feel loved and a daughter who only wanted to feel loved, now just two women sharing a deep loss and feeling a common heartache.

II.
The Stranger Who
Used to Be My Mother:
1999

In Over His Head

When my father was five, his father walked him to the end of a pier, then picked him up and threw him into the ocean. The water smacked and surprised Paul. Waves surrounded and sucked at him. He splashed his arms, opened his mouth, coughed, swallowed, and somehow managed to stay afloat until he was washed to shore.

His father was waiting on the beach for him, ready to wrap a towel around him and dry him off. "Good work, Pablo," he said softly. "I knew you had it in you."

According to my father, this was one of his first lessons in determination and problem solving.

My Aunt Ethel smiles when I tell her this story. In her early nineties, she has the manner of a genteel fairy with a slightly naughty past. Her fierce red hair frames her sweet, pale face. Her black dress, hose, and shoes are set off by a simple necklace of pearls.

"Actually, Papa threw him into a lake," she says. "At least that's the way I remember it. That was the way of Papa; he loved to prove that he was in control."

"But wasn't he teaching Dad about determination and problem solving?" I ask, sipping tea and resisting yet another of those delicious sugary wafers she has stacked on a china plate.

"That is the gift of your father—he has always taken what life threw him into, and learned from it."

When my father was first thrown into confusion by my mother's seemingly persistent passive-aggressive behavior, her inability to concentrate, and stubborn lack of memory, once again, he felt as though he were drowning. He splashed his arms and opened his mouth, coughed, swallowed, and looked toward the shore. Someone had moved the shoreline. Someone had moved anything resembling *terra firma*. There was my mother, staring defiantly ahead, refusing to remember where they were going, refusing to talk with him about the cruise they had taken five years ago, unwilling to apologize for the argument they had had the evening before. Here was the woman he loved, who had recently hidden his mail, put his dirty laundry in the garbage can, and burnt their brand-new teapot. Once again, Pablo was in over his head.

The Black Hole

My father is now living with a stranger, a woman he does not know or understand. He is afraid to go to sleep, because she wanders around at night. She, who cannot remember what a can opener, an avocado, or a shoelace is, has figured out how to unlock the apartment door, find the elevator, press the down button, get in, and wander out through the lobby. The guard on duty quickly retrieves her, but her unchecked mobility unnerves my father.

And last night, she urinated on the floor. My father called me at 10:30 p.m. in a panic.

"Why would she do that?" My father can barely speak, he is so distraught. "It's so immodest, so unlike her. Is it because we moved? Do you think she's trying to get back at me for moving us to Kansas City?"

"It's the disease," I say. "Do you want me to come and help you clean up?"

I realize my father has never changed a diaper, never dealt with this type of intimacy. Though he has valiantly accepted so many changes in my mother, this latest change screams at him, "She is ill. You cannot take care of her." This loss of bladder control announces she is no longer the clean, thoughtful woman he has loved all these years.

We go to the Alzheimer's Association for counseling and support. The social worker serves us coffee and cookies, gives Mom a book of photographs to look through, and shows us pictures of the brain with Alzheimer's. I have seen this before in textbooks, but I have never seen the blackened, blank area so large, so real, so linked to someone I love. The social worker is trying to show my father that this is not Mom's fault. Mom is not being churlish, wicked, or mean. She has fallen into the black hole in her own brain and is moving through space with very few anchors.

We listen as the social worker describes the progression of the disease. I think of a clearance sale, the sign that announces, *Everything Must Go*. As she talks, I look at Mom, patiently turning pages. Everything Must Go; I try to understand my mother will lose everything: Her legs will be capable of walking, dancing, and running, but her brain will not have the consciousness to move them. Her arms will be strong enough to rise up, to bend, to wiggle, but her mind will not allow the movement of the fork to her mouth. She will lose one function after another, until she is a mere rag doll.

The social worker closes the book of Alzheimer's brains. Then she looks at us carefully and says, "Meanwhile, the trick is to enjoy and care for Frances as she is right now. She has plenty of life left in her, and you want to make the most of that."

My father stares at Mom, who seems pleasantly occupied with her pictures. The last month has been a time of extraordinary change and loss for my father. My parents gave up their home in Memphis, where they lived for almost fifty years. They moved to a Kansas City retirement community. And now, my father finds himself in close quarters with a woman who is lewd and crazy.

Perhaps he is asking God, "Why, why, why?" Perhaps he is screaming inside, "NOOOOOO!" My own emotions are swirling. I can't stand to believe those pictures and that disease progression have anything to do with my mother—or with me.

A gripping fear whispers, "This disease can be hereditary, and whatever happens to my mother could happen to me." I want to run out of the building and separate myself from my mother.

The social worker touches my arm. "We have wonderful support groups," she tells me. I nod numbly.

"You both are doing an excellent job of coping with this," she says.

I look at Dad to see if he's going to mention the loss of bladder control. He is carved into an unmoving portrait of sorrow. I quietly mention that issue, and the social worker nods. "It's a natural part of the process," she says. "Are you considering a nursing home?"

Again I look at my father, but he cannot speak; he is immobilized by the black-and-whiteness of those terrible photographs.

I nod. "We are starting to consider that."

"Let me give you some guidelines and suggestions," she says.

She recommends some assisted living facilities close to their retirement center. Mom stands up and walks over to Dad. He absently pats her arm. She touches his shoulder.

"I need the bathroom," she says.

I guide her to the bathroom. I wait outside for her, making sure the door is ajar, not locked. I hear a flush and wait for several minutes. Then I peek inside. Mom is standing in front of the sink, staring. I go in and turn on the water for her, show her the soap.

"They keep moving these things. I wish they wouldn't move them," she says. I can only imagine the puzzle of each ordinary daily activity.

Leaving the building, my father can barely move. His feet have grown heavy in the last hour, his arms leaden. I open the car door for him, and he practically falls into the backseat.

"Why don't I take you home, Dad? Mom and I will have a little outing," I offer.

He nods.

I understand what he's feeling. Somehow all the information, all the fears, all the material we've heard and read about Alzheimer's have come together in one no-nonsense, irrefutable piece. All our excuses, our conjectures, our hoped-for cures have been smashed, at least temporarily, and we are facing a stark reality.

"Paul, are you all right?" Mom says as Dad gets out of the car and heads into the retirement community.

He turns and I see the tears trailing down his cheeks.

"Yes, darling, I'm fine. I'm just tired. I'm going to rest while you and Debbie go out and have some lunch."

"Okay, darling. See you soon."

He creates a quick smile. "Yes, soon."

I pull away and Mom says, "Is he all right?"

"He's just worried about you," I tell her. "He'll be all right."

"I hope so," she says.

I am touched by my mother's concern. My own concern for my father helps me pull myself together. Right now, it's just me and my mother, going out to lunch.

I am on alert to make the lunch easy and stress-free for her. I unwrap her silverware, so the closed-up white napkin won't confound her. I quickly scan the menu, so I can tell her what she might like, giving her two choices. Then I order for her, so she won't have to lose a sentence and get that anxious look on her face. I remove the container of salad dressing, so she won't drink it. I open the packet of cream and pour it into her coffee. I watch to see if she needs any help buttering her roll. I pat her hand as she gratefully says, "Thank you, darling," trying to forget that she is calling me darling because she does not remember my name.

Soon after Mom and I have returned to my house, my father calls.

"How is everything?" he asks.

"Fine. We're just hanging out. Take your time."

"I'm ready to come get your mother," he tells me.

"Dad's going to be here soon," I tell Mom. I feel her relax. Perhaps she was worried he would abandon her, not love her anymore. Perhaps she knows how different she is and wonders if he can take it.

When Dad arrives, his face is softened. My mother has always been the one in charge of any emotional crisis. But now, she is the cause of the crisis. My father looks at me in a new way. We are partners, a team working on behalf of my mom.

"I missed you," Mom says as he tenderly leads her to the car.

Now I am the one to sit numbly and stare into space. I look around my living room and imagine a man walking in and silently removing the sofas. No comfortable way to sit down. Another man comes in and takes the coffee table. No place to set down a teacup. One person removes the pictures and lamps, another hauls out the books. I imagine the room stripped down to its original emptiness.

"My mother is going to lose everything," I say aloud, hearing my voice echo in the imaginary emptiness.

The invisible men will take all the knowledge, information, connections, jokes, love of art and color, friends, joy in family, recipes, all the things that made her into mother, wife, and friend. She will be a string of missing objects and lost functions. I sit unmoving, my heart locked, my brain cold. A wave of anguish starts in my belly and howls into my mouth. The sound is too raw, too primitive to come from me, and I put my hands over my lips, then bite down on my fingers. The snap of pain, the nip of my teeth against my hands steadies me.

I remember walking into my house before I bought it and falling in love with the emptiness, the scarred wooden floors, the wide-open space, and the plain, cream-colored walls. Even without any of the comfort and familiarity of furniture, the rooms had their own beauty.

I close my eyes and imagine that beauty. I pray I will have the courage to discover who my mother is, day by day, and to love her as her new emptiness unfolds.

The Tease

On my mother's first day in assisted living, she causes a little stir in the activities room.

In that beautifully furnished, deeply carpeted room, with its round tables and comfortable chairs, twenty people are gathered to create necklaces. Bright plastic beads are piled in the center of each table. Mom and I sit together, like two kids, making a necklace. Or rather, I am creating the necklace: Mom restlessly hums and looks around.

This is the first time Mom has ever been separated from my father. A mere three months after their move to Kansas City, and Dad can no longer take care of her in their retirement-home apartment—her wandering, her confusion, her all-night wakefulness, and her incontinence have turned dangerous. She leaves the stove on and the door to the apartment open; she walks out of the building in the middle of the night. Even though assisted living is only one step up from the retirement center, our decision to place her in this home is wrenching. We are simmering with guilt and worried about her feeling abandoned, confused, and unloved. There is not much we can do about her confusion—she is already wading deeper into Alzheimer's—but Dad and I decide to take turns being with her during these first difficult days.

As I happily create a necklace, Mom gets up and wanders to the center of the room. I figure she is going to mingle and talk with people; she has a social nature, and I am pleased she is going to make friends. But I am not pleased when I look up to see Mom blithely unbuttoning her blouse, a naughty little smile lighting up her face.

"Mom!" I say, but before I can stop her, she has dropped her blouse to the ground. Her smile grows bigger. I rush up to her, as does one of the aides. The aide takes off her lab coat and covers Mom up, clasping Mom's hand before she can slip down her bra straps.

"Mom, you can't do that," I say as we escort my mother back to her room.

"I can," Mom says, with a little-girl sparkle to her voice.

Once Mom has another shirt on, I walk her to the small dining room, where we have juice and cookies together. We look through a magazine and she seems herself again, disconnected from the everyday world, but still able to sometimes tell a story about her old life. She is happy to see me and wonders where Dad is.

Dad wonders where she is when he comes to visit the next afternoon. She is not in her room, the activity room, or the dining room.

"They often go into other patients' rooms," an aide explains, and together they walk down the corridors looking for Mom. They find her asleep on the single bed of George G. Walsh. Mr. Walsh is rummaging through his dresser when my father walks in. In other circumstances it might have looked compromising, and to my father it still looks rather shady. Mr. Walsh is a good-looking older gentleman. He is tall, with a wonderful wealth of white hair (my father puts his hand to his own nearly naked scalp) and wearing a nice sport shirt and rather stylish-looking khaki pants, bought within at least the last year. My father feels the shabbiness of his own wrinkled white shirt and his slacks, bought at least three decades earlier in a discount department store on Memphis's Beale Street.

"Frances, get up. You don't belong in this room," my father says.

"She can stay as long as she likes," Mr. Walsh intones. His voice, as my father must note, is deep and articulate, deeper even than my father's own excellent voice.

The aide is waking Mom up.

"This is my wife," my father says, forgetting he is standing in an assisted living facility and that Mr. Walsh might not be the Casanova that he seems. "She does not belong here. Frances, come on," Dad says while putting his arm about Mom, and with the aide helping her to her feet.

"Are you insulting me?" Mr. Walsh demands, walking right up to my father, readying his fists. He is tall, and now that he is so close, Dad is pretty sure he is strong as well.

The nurse aide pushes between them. "Come on, George," she says pleasantly, "Let's go have a cup of coffee and find you the newspaper."

George follows her, but not before he has sent Dad a black glare. Dad hurries Mom back to her room, lecturing all the way on the perils of strange men.

"Yes, dear," my mother says, in the tone that means she knows something important is being said but she has no idea what.

I have often wondered about my mother's sexual past, something she never revealed to me except to laugh about her string of beaus named Harry. Mom always seemed so prudish. She and Dad seldom embraced in front of us when we were growing up. She always wore modest clothes and disapproved of those who flaunted their charms. And yet, when I was thirteen and looking in her bedside table for a photo album, I discovered a tattered copy of *Lady Chatterley's Lover.*

The next day, when I walk into my mother's room, Mom is sitting on her bed, looking through a picture album, and Mr. Walsh is rifling through my mother's underwear drawer.

"Excuse me," I say to him, but Mr. Walsh does not stop his activities.

I help Mom up and walk her to one of the lounges. On the way, I tell a nurse about Mr. Walsh, and she promises to keep him out of Mom's room.

Dad and I have been duly warned about changes in Mom's behavior, but the warnings were focused on forgetfulness, wandering, inattention, and sudden bouts of aggression and sleeplessness. Nobody mentioned stripping, sleeping in other men's beds, or letting a man rummage through her lingerie.

Who is this woman I am walking with? Is this her true nature, coming out now that she is less burdened with modesty and decorum? Or is this some intangible collapse of synapses, the crushing of a well-traveled neural path? Is this a last act of defiance in a prim and proper life, or a simple stumble?

For two weeks, Mom continues to wander into Mr. Walsh's room; undress randomly in the dining room, corridor, and activity room; and spread her underwear on her bed or on her floor. My father and I worry about her dignity and her safety. We don't know what to do or how to help her.

And then, as suddenly as it started, the sexual revolution is over. My mother stops unbuttoning her blouse. If she wanders into somebody else's room, she fiddles with the closet doors and the toiletries around the sink, but avoids the beds. She forgets where her underwear drawer is. Her naughty smile is replaced by a calmer one. Perhaps it has been her way of having a last unruly fling. Perhaps it is just part of the disease.

I remember that defiant, sexy sparkle in her eyes as she let her blouse fall to the ground, as if to say, "Try and stop me. Try and stop any of this."

And, of course, we simply can't.

In the Eyes of the Beholders

The staff at assisted living has Mom ready, just as I asked. I take Mom's hand and say, "Come on. This is going to be fun."

My smile says we are going to fly kites or eat banana splits. She follows me, a slight drag to her step. I open the car door and remind her to sit down. I have to press on her shoulder so she remembers what to do. I drive carefully, watching to make sure she is not fiddling with the locks. The last time we went out, she got the door open while we were driving. Dad fell apart when he heard about it. "Do you think she's trying to commit suicide?" he wanted to know.

"An adventure," I say, swinging Mom's hand as we walk into the beauty salon. The woman directs me to three pink, vinyl-covered chairs and a glass-top table that holds a well-worn copy of *People* magazine and a large, thick hardback called *Style*. I guide Mom to a chair and open the big book. Each page gleams with a large picture of a pixie, a vixen, or a sexy siren, viewed from the neck up. One has moussed hair that looks like the prow of a ship. Another has curls as still as marble, and another's hair waves as if she's in a wind tunnel. I hold the book close to Mom and point at each picture. She likes pictures.

We have looked through all the books, and I can feel Mom getting restless. At the nursing home, Mom has refused to bathe, refused to let them wash her hair or trim her fingernails. "She gets combative," the nurse told me. "We've got to let her get past this." My father went to intervene—he would bathe her himself. But Mom fought him as well.

Meanwhile, her hair has grown long and greasy, her nails are gnarled and yellowed. She looks like the crone in the old fairy tales, the kind of witch who will take bread and water you offer and in return for your kindness give you a valuable secret that might save your life. Much as I enjoy fairy tales, I want Mom to look like her normal, clean and groomed self again, not like some hideously disguised fairy-tale villainess. Her unkempt hair and unchecked fingernails make me feel sad and ashamed. How can I let my mother look so dirty and forgotten?

"Frances?" A stocky woman wearing a green smock over black pants stands before us. "I'm Kim. Pleased to meet you."

I take Mom's hand and lead her to a chair in the center of a long row. I hold her hands while Kim puts a smock over her.

"So how do you want it cut?" Kim asks.

Mom is swiveling in the chair.

"She usually wears it short," I say. "We need to be quick, because I don't know how long she will last."

Kim nods and gets out her scissors.

I kneel and hold Mom's hands. Mom smiles. Locks of her silvery hair float down and come to rest at my feet. Mom has always been her own barber, until last year, when scissors no longer made any sense.

This is only Mom's second time ever in a beauty parlor. The first time was when her niece got married and all the women went together to get fancy hairdos. My mother got her first dose of rollers, hair dryers, and hairspray. And she was introduced to the idea of protecting hair, like it was an endangered species, wrapping toilet paper around the set so it wouldn't deflate during careless sleep. But before the night was over, Mom tore off the toilet tissue and splashed water on her bouffant hairdo, recapturing her familiar curls.

I sit on the floor, hold Mom's hands, and talk to Kim about her grandchildren. The hair blankets my legs and the floor. I have never knelt before my mother, and it seems like I should be saying, "Thank you for birthing me, for raising me, for being such an interesting and constant person in my life." It seems I should be thanking her for my very being, instead of saying to Kim, "Let's try to wash her hair while we're here."

We lead her to the sink. Mom giggles when Kim sprays warm water on her head, then lathers. Kim is quick, and when Mom emerges she looks like the woman I know, clean, with glorious, naturally curly hair.

"Is there a manicurist available who could do Mom's nails very quickly?" I ask.

Isabelle is available. She speaks with a soft Spanish accent. I sit right beside Mom as Isabelle puts Mom's hands in soaking water, and then shows her the selection of nail polish colors. Mom picks up a bright-red bottle, one that a younger Mom would have warned me against for being too bold. But when you're in your eighties, you can be bold. Mom clutches the bottle in one hand, refusing to let go of it, so Isabelle works on Mom's other hand, using a similar color. Mom watches for a while. When it's time, she unfurls her fingers and Isabelle quickly transforms the other hand.

In her real life, my mother never had her fingernails polished. She thought it vain and unnecessarily flirtatious. Perhaps she would still think that now. But that simple sparkle of color and elegance adds to Mom's presence, giving her an extra vibrancy.

"I add some lipstick and blush. Your mother, she is a beautiful woman," Isabelle says.

Years ago, when my aunt became feeble, her one despair was that she couldn't make it to her hairdresser, who lived across town.

"Why don't you go to the salon in your neighborhood?" I had asked Aunt Ann. "It's so much easier and closer."

"It's not the same. I'm used to my hairdresser."

Every week, I drove her to the hairdresser. Though I saw how happy she was, emerging with her hair newly set and tinted, her nails glowing pink, and her lipstick freshened, I still did not understand how being coifed and groomed could make such a difference.

Until now.

Now that Mom looks like she used to, I feel a sense of ease and hope. The dread of seeing Mom with dirty, old-woman hair melts away. Back at my house, we sit on the sofa and I hand her a cookie that I had stashed in my pocket, ready to bribe her into stillness if needed. She holds it like it is jewelry she doesn't own. "It's to eat," I tell her, moving her hand toward her mouth.

"Where is?" Mom can't find the next word, but I know she is asking about my dad.

"He'll be here in about an hour," I tell her.

We eat cookies and look at pictures in magazines. It feels like an after-school ritual with a beloved child.

When my father arrives, his eyes fill with tears when he sees Mom's hair. "What happened?" he asks. "Did you get her to take a bath?" His voice is low and awestruck.

"We went to the beauty parlor."

We look at her as if she is a brand-new person, pretty and full of possibility. Maybe this means she will be able to button her clothes again, remember my daughters' names, and recognize a Hershey's bar. Maybe something else will change. For these few moments, we believe anything is possible.

Love in the Land of Dementia

"There's my man," my mother says to the nurse, beaming at my father. He has been out of the room for five minutes, but Mom greets him like he has been gone for days.

Shyly, my father comes up to her and takes her hand. They look at each other.

"Fifty-two years married," my father tells the nurse as she checks the IV.

She shakes her head. "And still in love," she marvels. She adjusts her blond ponytail, pulls the stethoscope out of the pocket of her smock, and leans over to listen to Mom's heart.

"Your main man, huh?" she says to Mom.

Mom smiles, making a noise right out of a Donald Duck cartoon. Then Mom picks up a corner of her hospital gown and tugs at it. She pleats it into little sections and tugs again. "Well, you so-and-so," she says to the gown. "If you aren't going to cooperate, you can't come with me."

I hand her a blanket. "Here," I say. She stares into the blanket like there's a child cradled inside. "What a sweet baby," she says. "I love you, baby."

I look at Dad, who shrugs and smiles.

Maybe this is the lesson we are all to learn eventually. In the end, only love is left.

With Mom's advancing Alzheimer's, much has been lost. Rising up and sitting down are complicated feats of gymnastic skill. All foodstuffs are foreign substances. Dressing, conversing, bathing, teeth brushing—all the events of everyday life are neatly erased from Mom's scope.

But when my dad walks in, for a moment she remembers this is her husband. For those seconds, happiness floods her.

"I wish I had a relationship like you two have," the evening nurse says wistfully. She's a thin, vigorous brunette from Dubuque, Iowa. She's already been through two husbands, she tells us as she gently wraps the blood pressure cuff around Mom's arm. "Neither one of them was worth the polish on my toenails," she says.

My parents don't have the perfect romance. Most of the time, Mom doesn't know Dad's there. Most of the time, he has to stand right in front of her to talk. Most of the time, Mom is her own entertainment center, bouncing off his words but not truly interacting with him.

But when he first enters the room, light fills her face. Her eyes are luminous and her silvery hair seems to glow. The distracted, anxious look leaves her and there's an angelic purity to her expression. For that moment, she is present and filled with love.

All who see this look—the certified nurse aide, the registered nurse, the lab tech, the social worker—respond with awe and envy. They coo and sigh. "Ahhh," they murmur, "that's the way it is supposed to be."

Even the doctor glances up from his clipboard, as if there's been an alien sighting. When he continues his charting, I wonder if he will write, "Patient exhibits symptoms of deep dementia and signs of true love." I wonder how far apart these two conditions are.

"I want you to kill me if I ever have to go into a nursing home," my mother used to say when she was about my age. "I want to die if I lose my mind."

According to her diagnosis, my mother has officially "lost her mind." She came to the hospital from an assisted living facility. The "worst," as she then envisioned it, has happened.

Does she want to die? I wonder as I watch Mom pick at the lint on her blanket. She is not "herself"; she is not the mother I have known and the wife Dad has loved. But despite all the losses, she is still someone well worth being around. Her greatness remains in this simple gift she shows us: When all the ordinary things are gone, the spirit can still remain. Love doesn't necessarily conquer anything or all, but it can outlast the rational parts of life.

Tomorrow, everything could change. My dad could walk in and Mom might not ever look up from her pleating, plucking, and picking. She might stare at him like she sometimes stares at me, knowing he's a nice person but not knowing just who he is.

But we no longer think of tomorrow. We are happy at the fact that Mom laughs, even if it's at a bowl of vanilla pudding. We are thrilled with the fact that she talks, even if she's addressing invisible children in a language that makes Pig Latin seem scholarly. And we are awed by the fact that she loves.

"So where's your husband?" the nurse aide asks as she organizes Mom's dinner tray.

Mom doesn't answer; she examines the pink plastic bracelet on her left wrist.

"Let's scoot up in the bed," the aide says. Mom doesn't move. She fiddles with the plastic.

Then Dad walks into the room. He stops in front of the bed. Mom stops fiddling. She looks at him and smiles. "My husband," she says in an awestruck voice. "My husband's here," she says to the nurse and to me.

"That's right," Dad says. I hear the joy and anguish in his voice. I hear the depth of his grief and the strength of his love.

Finding the Key

She wanders around all night and sleeps all day. She grabs onto objects and won't let go. She won't sit on the toilet, won't keep on her diaper, and won't be given a bath. She talks to invisible, miniature men who live on the floor.

My father and I are devastated, embarrassed, and confused by Mom's aberrant and asocial behavior.

"We just can't take care of her," the administrator of assisted living tells us at yet another family meeting. "The doctor recommends you take her to the geriatric ward at the psych hospital. They can adjust her medications so she's more comfortable and more manageable. Then we'll be able to take care of her here."

"Maybe I could talk to her one more time," Dad says.

"She can't help herself, Mr. Barnett. It's the disease."

The geriatric psych ward occupies the fourth floor of a nearby medical center. We have to check in through the emergency room, and I am worried the chaos and frantic activity will unsettle Mom. I pack magazines, photographs, and cookies to help us through the time. Mom seems unaware of her setting. She plays with the buttons on her shirt, and she won't give up her coat.

After we have waited for a long time, a nurse ushers us to a small room for an EKG, blood work, temperature, blood pressure, and other tests.

A young doctor breezes through and says, "Her blood work is gorgeous."

An EMT-in-training stands around and tells us his life story: how his dad was no good and his uncle raised him, how he made straight A's in school and now is going to be an EMT, how he works nights as a bartender. We listen, happy to be distracted as we wait, endlessly it seems, for Mom to be admitted.

Mom's room is in a locked ward. No memory boxes with family photos here, no cheerful reality-orientation calendars reminding us of month and day, no crayon drawings from caring kindergarteners; just names on the doors, with the nursing instructions "Push fluids, soft diet, exercise daily."

I imagine writing "Feed ice cream" on Mom's door. It's one of the only things she still likes to eat.

The first two days, Mom is alert, as usual. She laughs with us when we visit, even though she is laughing at little men on the shiny linoleum floor instead of at my father's jokes.

She eats the bananas and candy my father brings. She says words.

Three days later, we find her conked out in a chair in the dining room.

"Hi, Mom. Hi, Frances. Hi, Fran," I say, touching her arm. No response.

My father says, "Hi, darling," his voice quavering.

Mom's hands flutter; her right leg rises up. Her eyes are closed. She is locked in some internal space. Our voices, our hands, our presence are not enough to bring her back.

"I think the medication is too strong," one nurse tells us. "The doctor will fix it tomorrow."

I ask if she can lay Mom down. Mom looks so uncomfortable, like a child fallen into slumped-over sleep. Two nurses get Mom into bed. My father and I stand on either side of her. She rouses for a moment, looks at me, looks at my father, gives him a little smile, then fades away again.

"I can't stand it that my mother has to go through all this," I tell Ron that night. I am pacing, the sadness and frustration of the situation gnawing at me. "Mom would hate this. She would hate being this drugged. Plus my father is so depressed and worried."

"It's natural for your dad to be worried," Ron says gently. "You can't stop his grief."

My mother has always been the emotional one. I am not used to seeing my father express feelings. His usual confident personality and the sense of showmanship that have made him so popular are gone. My heart aches for my father, and I yearn to comfort him. But he turns his head when he cries and won't let me stay in the room.

For three days, my mother is in a deep, drugged fog. The doctor comes by while Dad and I are talking to her, hoping our voices will sink into her, that she will feel our love and concern.

"She should be more alert," the doctor says. "This is the same dosage I gave her yesterday. She should be more alert." He leans against the wall, looking puzzled.

"What is she taking?" I ask. He gets the chart, and my father and I look at each other.

With the chart in hand, the doctor is more confident. He sits beside us and explains his priorities: noncombativeness, sleeping at night, eating, alertness, and freedom from hallucination.

"She's been hallucinating a lot, and I was trying to get rid of that for her," he says.

"We'd rather she be alert. If she has to hallucinate, that's okay. She seemed cheerful when she was hallucinating," I tell him.

"All right," he agrees. "This is all such experimentation. It's a delicate balance to get the highest quality of life. Then, three months go by, the disease progresses, and you have to start all over again."

I try not to see my father's face when he hears those words. I try not to imagine the ache in his heart.

I make friends with the nurses.

"I don't think this combination of medications is working for Mom," I say quietly. "What do you think we should try next?"

I want my mother back. I WANT my mother back! is what I'm really saying.

The nurses always have ideas. I share their ideas with the doctor. He listens, nods.

"We could try that," he says. I am grateful for his flexibility. I realize no one really knows what to do. Drug interaction is uncertain enough with a healthy brain; combined with Alzheimer's, it's like playing roulette.

For several days, I make myself do my work, visit Mom, and talk to Dad. I pack my sorrow away. I find it at night, when I tell Ron about Mom. The more I say about Mom, the more my voice dissolves. Soon, I am crying. I am howling. The loss of her, which has been so gradual, is now too large to think about. Ron takes me onto his lap. "Yes, cry," he soothes.

I cry. I lie against him and give up everything. I have no mother, no self, nothing but pure emptiness. I fall asleep, and when I wake up I am my mother's daughter once again, strong, capable, able to solve tall problems in a single bound.

"She's so drugged she can't walk," I tell the doctor the next day. I let my voice rise, but I'm not nearly as loud as I'd like to be.

"It takes a while to get the correct dosage," he says.

"She's been here ten days," I remind him.

"Every patient is different in the way he or she responds to the drugs. We can't predict how long it will take."

I call the social worker at the Alzheimer's Association.

"She's so drugged she can't walk. She can't feed herself," I say, trying to muffle my tears.

"Those drugs are tricky," she says. "Maybe you can find a place that will take your mother even if she's acting out. She may need a greater level of care than assisted living."

"Will you help us?"

Dad and I visit the home the social worker suggests, hesitating before we enter the locked Alzheimer's unit. At assisted living, I can pretend I am visiting Mom at some low-key resort. The warm-colored carpeting, thick early-American-style furniture, and the hallways with Impressionist posters promise "everything will be all right."

But once we push the red button and the door opens into the no-nonsense atmosphere of an Alzheimer's unit, there are no false promises. A wiry, bent-over woman strides the hallway, stopping only to bang her fist against the wall. A wild-looking, gray-haired man resists a nurse aide, shouting, "I am waiting for my wife. My wife will be here any minute. Mary, where are you?"

"Where do I go?" a sweet-looking woman in a forest-green pants suit asks as we tentatively step inside. "Where do I go? Do you know?"

Another grandmotherly type pauses in the hallway to tug down on her black slacks. A nurse aide rushes over and pulls the slacks back up.

Only weeks ago, I would have shied away from this kind of loud, expressive atmosphere. Now I am comforted by it. There is plenty of chaotic, aberrant, asocial behavior going on: Mom can fit right in.

The head nurse nods calmly as Dad and I tell her about Mom's behavior. "We can handle it," she says. "Just know that it's not going to stop right away. Don't be mad at us if she continues to act out for a while."

When they moved from Memphis to Kansas City, Mom and Dad required a moving van, four strong men, and two agile boys to move her possessions. Then four of us spent two full days unpacking, getting her and Dad settled in their retirement-community apartment. Now, a nurse aide pushes a wheelchair draped with Mom's clothes. Dad and I each carry a grocery sack full of underwear and socks. The move is eerily simple. And it could have been simpler still, if we'd have been willing to give up the clothes she can no longer wear: her once-favorite blouses, dresses, and slacks that require hooks, zippers, and buttons. Mom is beyond all fastening devices.

Two days ago, Dad and I brought some of Mom's things to her new room, to make it cozy and familiar. Still, when we walk in today, it's strange to see family pictures already set up on the bedside table. A pillow wearing one of Mom's familiar cases rests on the blue-ribbed bedspread. An afghan that a friend crocheted covers the bottom half of the bed.

A woman wearing a pink sweatsuit and bunny slippers shuffles into the room and touches Mom's hair. Mom doesn't seem to notice. The woman fingers the fabric of Mom's sweatshirt, picks at the cuff, and then shuffles off.

Dad hands Mom a picture of my brother and me when we were little. She takes it, but doesn't look at it. She is staring into some private world, still lost in a medicated stupor.

A man in green scrubs comes in, the assistant director of nursing.

"She was a World War II nurse," Dad tells him.

"I was in a MASH unit in 'Nam. We've seen some things, haven't we dear?" he says to Mom.

She just stares. I hang up clothes Mom will never wear, pretty clothes that are too awkward to dress her in.

An aide comes in and helps Mom into bed. Once Mom lies down, she is fast asleep.

"Okay," Dad says, "we can go now. I'll come back tonight."

The nurse aide tells us the secret code we must punch in to leave the unit.

"Some of the residents may try to get out if you open the door too wide," she says. "Just be careful when you leave."

I feel like a spy as I look around, and then stealthily punch in the code. A green light blinks, a latch clicks. We push open the door and close it carefully behind us.

For a week, Mom remains in the medicated haze. Then I begin to see small signs of emergence. She starts to walk again, though she moves slowly in a shuffle. She notices the little men on the linoleum floor and says a word or two to them. She laughs a couple of times, at nothing.

During the second week of Mom's stay at the Alzheimer's unit, the nurse stops me in the hall when I come to visit.

"She started to take down her pants and urinate in the hallway," she says. "We caught her just in time."

"Thanks," I say.

I hide my smile.

She's back, I think. My embarrassing, terrible, antisocial mother has returned.

I can't wait to see her.

The Tribe

Some people walk into the Alzheimer's unit and see a bunch of addled old ones, like loony, lonely fairy princesses, roaming the hallways. Some people see great men and women reduced to remnants, scraps of their former selves. I walk in and see the community in this corridor, a tribe of people strangely united.

It is surprising to think of these disparate individuals, adult diapers bulging under sweatpants, walking with one sock and one black tennis shoe, as having a common thread. They rarely talk to each other; if one speaks, the other seldom creates a coherent answer. They do not look or smile at each other as they pass in the hallway. In the Alzheimer's unit the tribal connection is intuitive, cellular, beyond the easily discernible.

I am first introduced to the notion of the tribe one day when I am sitting on a blue chair in the dining room, watching my mother eat her lunch. Anna, a crusty, iron-haired woman, says to the nurse, "Dammit, Kelly, I want to go to my room and I want to go now."

"Anna, you can't talk that way in the dining room," Kelly says firmly. Normally Kelly is as smooth and sweet as creamery butter. Now, her tone is unusually tough-sounding.

As Kelly puts Mom's dessert cup in front of her, she leans over and whispers to me, "If I let Anna talk that way, soon they'll all start cursing. The families will get upset."

I look at each person, some eating with spoons, some scarfing food with their hands, some staring, others resting their heads on the table. I can't imagine them behaving as a group.

"It's true. It's happened several times and it really gets out of hand quickly," Kelly says.

As if to illustrate, Fred, who has been resting at the table, raises his head and says, "Poop." Ida, dimple-faced in pink sweats, rolls her walker by and shouts, "Phooey on you." Mom looks up from chasing a kernel of corn with her spoon and says, "Criminy."

The rampage has begun.

"Not in here, Fred," Kelly insists. "Ida, you'll have to go to your room if you keep that up."

I look around, wondering if anyone really understands Kelly. No one nods, yet somehow, the rebellion ends.

The tribe has no formal ceremonies or rites, no inner circles or talking sticks. But tonight, I can feel something is wrong. Mom fiddles with her sleeve instead of eating her mashed potatoes. Nancy's hands flutter so badly that her spoon flies to the floor. Helen, usually an avid eater, merely picks at her meat loaf with a manicured finger. At first, I think the moon is too full or the coffee too strong. Then I notice that Mildred is not in the dining room. Mildred graces every meal with her amazing Hepburnesque beauty and her high voice, repeating, "I want to go home. Take me home. I'm cold. Take me home." Mildred only eats her dessert and always looks elegant in her Irish wool sweaters and pleated slacks. Mildred is the *Vogue*, the *Elle*, the *Women's Wear Daily* in this land of mismatched socks and appliquéd sweatshirts.

"Where's Mildred?" I ask Kelly, who's working a double shift.

"She had to go the hospital. She was dehydrated and spiked a fever we couldn't bring down," Kelly answers. She leans over Helen and croons, "Are you eating today, Helen? Come on, I've got something you'll like." Kelly wiggles the spoon into the blended meat loaf and coaxes a bite into Helen's mouth, with the same tenderness with which she might feed her own child.

"Do you think they know?" I say, gesturing to the people in the dining room.

"They know," Kelly says. "They know one of their own has gone missing and they don't know what to do about it."

In a former time, in a former place, the tribe might go on a search, crying out, beating the brush, looking everywhere for the one gone missing.

Here, the residents walk the halls at night, some using walkers, others shuffling along on their own. They sit down in front of the television, 2:00 a.m., blinking at ancient reruns of *The Dating Game*. Then they walk again. They press against the unit's locked door, they mumble, they move on. In the morning, heads droop against the breakfast table. Brenda, the one with the foghorn voice, forgets to complain about her meal.

The tribe is uneasy. No one is capable of saying, "Where is Mildred? It feels strange without her." Their words come out in gestures and sounds: Their hands flutter; they mumble and jerk. Someone is lost, gone; there is emptiness, and the tribe feels it deeply.

I am not part of this tribe. Of course, I don't want to be. I celebrate my ability to walk out of the building, remembering how strong are my legs, how swift is my mind. I am a foreigner in this land. I have too much language, too much discernment, and too many manners to be absorbed into the group. So I am cast out of the emotional connection that wobbles and weaves, so invisible, so indistinguishable, and yet so deep.

Though this tribe has almost nothing, its members have something I want: a connection that goes beyond name, age, career, economics, and religion. They are part of something larger, deeper, and closer to God. I dread such closeness, such primal expressiveness, and yet I yearn for it. But that yearning is something I cannot speak. My normal, easy words seem so hollow and so aloof, so far away from what I am feeling.

Still, for now, those words are what I have. All I can do is wait until my next visit and ask in a casual voice, "How's Mildred coming along?"

III.
Hanging On to What Is Left:
SPRING 2000–2001

The Emblem

On October 10, 1948, my parents celebrated their wedding with a dinner for ten at the Palmer House, one of Chicago's elegant hotels. The cost of the dinner was $90. My father kept the receipt. Decades later, when he and Mom were going to celebrate their fiftieth wedding anniversary, he had a grand idea. We would all, my children and I, my brother and his family, meet in Chicago and stay at the Palmer House to celebrate the anniversary.

But the grand idea nearly got shattered after his first conversation with the hotel reservations clerk.

"Two hundred and fifty dollars a night." Dad's voice was subdued when he called to give me the discouraging news. "And that's with Triple-A and senior discounts. I'll have to think of something else."

He did. My father was an expert at the development and execution of the Grand Plan.

He decided to call the manager of the Palmer House and see if he wanted to put us all up for free, in honor of their anniversary and of the wedding dinner he had enjoyed so many years earlier. It would be great publicity for the hotel and great fun for all of us.

He called the hotel manager, who did not return his call.

He called again. No call back.

My father was a salesman, so this impolite behavior only fueled his determination.

He called the hotel manager's executive assistant and told her his story, using his deep radio voice, his eloquent vocabulary, and his humble-yet-irresistible charm.

"I'll see what I can do," she said.

She called back. She asked for a copy of the receipt for the original wedding meal. My father mailed it. She told my father she could offer him and his wife a complimentary suite on the penthouse floor for three days.

We were all ecstatic. The rest of us stayed in cheaper quarters nearby.

Every night, management sent up two bottles of fine champagne to my parents' suite. Every afternoon, they offered us all hors d'oeuvres in the penthouse lounge. They gave us a gift certificate for the anniversary dinner at the hotel dining room.

My mom and dad had a $1,000 weekend for free. It was a tribute to true love, persistence, creative thinking—and to saving your receipts forever.

That weekend, my mother was struggling with the confusion of early Alzheimer's. My dad was pretending nothing was amiss. But in the weeks to follow, when he could no longer deny the changes, he created a new form of the Grand Plan, a series of ideas, research projects, connections, and activities that would help my mother return to normal. It was a tribute to true love, persistence, creative thinking—and to saving your hope forever.

A Drop of Honey

Hours before our Rosh Hashanah dinner, I sit down at the kitchen table to write checks. While I write, I think of my rabbi friend Jeff, who is spending the week visiting elderly Jews in nursing homes.

"The Jewish New Year is a holiday of remembering both your sins and your blessings," Jeff had reminded me just last night.

Inside the hushed facilities smelling of tired chrysanthemums, meat loaf baking, and the entwined odors of urine and disinfectant, he walks to the end room of the green hallway, greeting residents as he goes. He closes the door to Mrs. Cohen's room behind him and sits beside her bed.

"Did you bring it?" she asks.

He opens his backpack and takes out the *shofar*, the ancient instrument that sounds on the New Year, announcing the ten-day period of prayer and atonement, the High Holy Days.

"Well then, let's hear it," Mrs. Cohen says.

Jeff stands, takes a deep breath, and blows. The sound, loud and unmelodic as a wounded animal, twists over the intercom announcements, over the sound of Bessie in the next room crying, "Help me, help me, help me," over the maintenance man buffing his way down the hallway. The *shofar* reminds us to return to God with humble spirit and to distinguish between the trivial and the important in life.

As I sit in my kitchen and write my checks, I think of that sound. I picture the rabbi of my childhood standing on the *bema* in his majestic black robes, blowing the *shofar*, the atonal sound like a soul struggling to rise above war and soar to victory.

I write one check to a charitable group that works with women who have been torn from their everyday lives, plunged into chaos, uprooted by war. I write to help a woman in Rwanda, one with six children and no shelter or food. I write to help a woman in Kosovo, a family in Bosnia. I write to help myself.

I write out another check, this one also to help those who have been torn from their everyday lives, plunged into chaos, uprooted, and forced to live in an alien world. I make the check out to an Alzheimer's research association. I write to save a friend's father. I write to save my mother. I write to save myself.

Ron has helped me prepare the holiday meal. His mother, Mollie, is the first to arrive. She bustles in carrying the chicken, kugel, and brownies she cooked up today. Her husband, Frank, walks more slowly behind her. Many people do not believe Mollie when she announces she is eighty-four years old. "Your skin is so smooth; you're so pretty, vibrant, and strong," they say.

Soon afterward, my father leads my mother into the house. Mom is having an evening away from the Alzheimer's unit. Her step is halting; she has the bewildered look of an astronaut who hasn't blasted off, yet somehow finds herself on the moon. She focuses on the tablecloth, which is silvery and full of sparkles. I hand her a glass of chardonnay, her favorite wine.

"What is this?" she asks. I tell her.

She takes an experimental sip and smiles. These days, Mom's life is like that trust-building exercise where you bond with a group of strangers, then fall backward into their waiting arms. For Mom, most everyone is now a stranger, and most every event, from eating to getting into the car to walking into this house, demands trust.

The aroma of Mollie's chicken envelops us. My daughters come in, fresh from work and working out, and we all gather at the table. Mollie lights the candles and blesses us in beautiful Hebrew. We begin passing around the food. My father serves my mother, her plate full of substances she has never seen before.

As our talk skids around from our daily lives to the local arts scene, I notice how protective my daughters are of their grandmother. They know not to embarrass her with a direct question, and yet they frequently smile at her and reach out to touch her hand. I wonder what it feels like to have their grandmother so changed. She has always loved them, but sometimes she was critical of my girls or their behavior. Her judgmental nature has melted away, and I see her sweetness now as she smiles at my children.

The candles flicker; we sip our wine. Then I slice an apple and say, "Take a piece and pour a drop of honey on it, to symbolize a sweet New Year."

Ever since I was a child, I have loved this part of the holiday, the ritual that isn't about sins and righteousness, but simply a reminder to choose a sweet life.

Dad hands Mom her apple. She examines the slice, oozing with honey, then shrugs. She's never seen such a thing before, but she's game. She bites into a fruit she's been eating for eighty-some years, a ritual she's been doing all her life, for the very first time.

Last night, my brother called from Tokyo. "I was finally able to cry," he told me. "I cried because the mother I know is gone. She has somehow disappeared."

I have cried, too. I have wrapped myself into a primal ball and wailed with the anguish of it all. "Poor Mom, poor Mom," I sobbed. I cried for my dad, who every day sees his lover, his soul mate, his companion become more of a child, more of a stranger, more of a burden. I cried for my brother, who cannot experience the losses gradually as I can, but who is shocked and startled by the changes he sees in Mom when he comes to visit. I cried for myself, the good daughter, the cheerful problem solver. I cried because I was sad, confused, tired, and scared. Scared that Alzheimer's would be hereditary, scared that this would happen to me.

"How are you holding up?" I asked my brother.

"Fair. This is all so unreal. When I called them last week, Mom didn't know who I was, didn't recognize my name, even after I told her I was her son." His voice cracked.

"She doesn't know who I am, most of the time," I told him. I let the piercing sadness of my sentence sink in: How could I be safe in the universe when my own mother, my sworn protector, did not recognize me?

I held the phone close to my ear, just feeling my brother's presence as we sat in silence for a moment, thousands of miles apart, feeling abandoned.

"So, how do you think Dad's doing?" Daniel asked, and we were back on easier, safer topics.

After I clear the table, I pull up a chair and sit beside Mom. She stumbles into talk. Most of her conversation is random phrases, remnants not even large enough for a handkerchief. I listen and remind myself, this is a time to remember blessings. Soon, even these stray syllables may go away. Then she says, "How is your mother?"

For a moment, I just look at her. I wonder who she sees when she looks at me. I smile and take her hands.

"Gosh, Mom, only you can answer that one," I cannot resist saying. "How *are* you?"

"Okay," she says, and we laugh.

The evening ends. I walk Mom out to Dad's car. I open the door, point her to the seat, and put on her seat belt. "It was fun," she says.

Three syllables. A complete sentence. A sentence of happiness, praise, and acknowledgment.

I walk back into the kitchen, the counters stacked with dirty dishes. One piece of apple, slightly browned, sits alone on a black plate. I hold the empty honey bear upside down to see if I can coax out one more drop. While I wait, I open the newspaper. A video store owner murdered just one mile from me. A woman kidnapped from a mall. A family who donated money to an animal shelter and saved the lives of hundreds of strays.

Every day there is war; every day there is victory. I squeeze the honey bear and wait; squeeze again; shake the bear. Nothing. Then I wait a moment longer and one drop falls onto the apple.

Once again, something to celebrate.

Bringing Magic to Life

When I come into the Alzheimer's unit, I hear Nat King Cole singing. I have to smile at the song "Unforgettable" being played in a place where so much has been forgotten.

My mother and many of the patients are gathered in the dining room for the afternoon activities. About eleven ladies and one man form a jagged circle in chairs. Arlene is laughing. Everyone else sits with bowed heads and solemn expressions, as if they were in the middle of a prayer service. I sit down beside my mother. A plastic box full of noisemakers is on her table. She fiddles with the lid.

"Hi, Mom," I say and I touch her arm. She keeps fiddling.

"Don't I know you?" Minnie asks me. She is sitting opposite Mom, holding a child's cymbal as if it were the top of a frying pan. She has the open, pleasant look of a backyard neighbor, one with an apple pie cooling and coffee brewing.

"You do know me," I say. "I'm Fran's daughter."

"It's too bad," she says. She continues, "I tarred we were going to, you know, but I guess I shouldn't ask about it, because, after all, they may schmletz it up, get mad, do you think?"

"We're going to exercise," says Rochelle, one of the afternoon aides. Rochelle has small braids that lie respectfully down her back. One gold tooth punctuates her wide smile. Her voice has an undertone of huskiness that sounds both sexy and inviting. Her voice makes people want to listen. Most people, that is.

George, one of the newer patients, has not yet been captured by Rochelle's voice. He does not seem inclined to join the circle. He has the air of a tired and retired poet, with his lean body, gentle stoop, and extravagant flop of white hair. In his jacket with the leather-padded elbows and his corduroy trousers, he looks like someone who would get out an ancient pipe and begin telling a long story. But George can barely get out a couple of words.

"Come on, George, sit down right here." Rochelle patiently guides him to a chair beside Judy, who is hunched over the baby doll she loves to carry.

Now Rochelle gets out a beach ball and begins tossing it around the circle. "Play ball, Arlene," she calls out cheerfully. Arlene can catch and throw back. Her husband was a college football star, and she scoops up the ball and tosses it across the circle. The ball flounders when it reaches Judy. Rochelle shows Judy the ball. Judy nods; she has stern gray hair and a determined New England air about her. She heaves the ball, and it thuds to a halt in the center of the small circle.

"Good job, Judy," Rochelle says and smiles at me. "Okay, Frances, it's your turn. Come on, Frances." Mom does not seem to notice the bright ball. She is bent over, rolling up the end of her sweater. When Rochelle hands her the ball, she clutches it and resumes her rolling.

"Mom was never very athletic," I tell Rochelle.

Elizabeth kicks the ball across the circle. Eudora examines it before she hands it back to Rochelle, as if it were a steak not cooked to order. George is holding a book, and won't let it go. Bill has fallen asleep.

Rochelle sticks in another tape, and soon "Stardust" is playing.

"Let's dance," she says, motioning everyone to stand up.

She reaches for Bonnie's hand, and she and Bonnie start to move together. Minnie gets up, as if she's wondering what to do. Arlene claps and laughs. Elizabeth and Eudora begin an awkward waltz together. Mom looks up, and I offer her my hand.

"Want to dance?" I ask her.

"What?"

"Want to dance?" I repeat, making a swirling motion.

"What else?" she says, standing up.

My parents have danced to this song many times, my mother coaxing my father onto the dance floor. I hold hands with Mom and move back and forth to the music. She laughs and does the same. I twirl her, and she walks around in a jaunty little circle. For a moment, her energy and charm have returned. I feel like I have found my long-lost mother. If my father were here, he would not be surprised. He is certain she will return to him and takes every word, every gesture of affection, every smile as a sign of hope.

"Hope is everything," Dad told me just last week. "I find something hopeful and I milk it for all it's worth. If it doesn't work out, then I search for something else. Otherwise, I am in despair."

I twirl my mom again. It is actually our first real dance together.

"Good job, Frances," Rochelle says.

"Wa wa wa," Mom says, like she is mimicking a cartoon character. She stands still, looks at her sweater, and picks at a loose thread. Her face is suddenly blank. Our dance is over.

Sally Jo walks in, on her usual route down the halls, in and out of every room. She spends her days with her head bent and her fists clenched, walking the unit endlessly, never stopping until someone leads her to a meal or a bath.

"Sally Jo used to be a dance instructor," Rochelle says. "Didn't you, Sally Jo?"

Sally Jo stops right in front of me and raises her head. Something secret flickers in her face. I look right at her. The secret light grows brighter. She unclenches her fists and turns a little from side to side. She smiles, and I realize how beautiful she is. I have rarely seen her smile; I have never seen her stop her walking. I keep looking into her eyes. She is glowing with inner fire. Then the song ends and Sally Jo bends her head and resumes her walking.

Mom returns to her chair.

"Red Sails in the Sunset" comes on. The kitchen aide wheels in a snack cart. Rochelle busies herself pouring milk and distributing cookies.

Everyone is back in their chairs, quiet, passive, their faces dim.

When I was a child, I was certain that my dolls were alive. They were just waiting for me to leave so they could laugh and talk to each other. I often dashed into my room to surprise them in their merriment, but I never caught them. Now I feel like I've finally entered that secret room, where the faces in the circle, all those beautiful, forgotten, aging dolls, come to life once again. Just for one moment, just for one dance.

Mom is involved with the cookie Rochelle handed out, too involved to acknowledge my hug good-bye. Sally Jo paces the halls. "Don't I know you?" Minnie asks as I wave good-bye. Everything seems normal once again, but I know better. I have seen the beauty of music and memories, and I am humming as I walk out.

An Ordinary Day

My mother is in her room in the Alzheimer's unit, lying abed, wearing a red, white, and blue pullover and an adult diaper. She is staring at two nurse aides who are holding her tennis shoes and a pair of red pull-on pants.

"Your mama is just getting up from her nap," the male aide says, his voice thick with a Jamaican accent.

Mom's hands are clasped and she's watching the proceedings as if this is the Entertainment Channel. I too am watching as the woman expertly pulls on Mom's pants. Part of me is thinking, I should be dressing my own mother, not having two strangers do the job. What kind of daughter am I that I just stand back and watch? But I am glad for their competent presence. I would be stymied by the immovability of my mother's hips and thighs—pushing her this way and that, inching the fabric upward. I would still be struggling with one pant leg on one passive calf. I would still be trying to coax that innocent and uncooperative foot into the yawning tennis shoe.

In only minutes, these two have quickly performed a task that seems daunting to me.

"Will you help me take her outside?" I ask.

Mom cannot stand on her own. The man holds her hands and she leans back, as if she were playing a game. She follows as he walks backward, guiding her through the corridor and out into the courtyard. The autumn weather is sweet and balmy.

Several of the other patients are already outside, Dorothy asleep on a chair next to us, Florence pacing, and Robert fiddling with a large potted tomato plant.

The aide sits Mom on a bench next to a yellow rosebush, and I sit down beside her. Our shoulders touch, like we are girlfriends sitting in the park, sharing confidences. I open the magazine I have brought and show Mom a picture of a boy eating blueberries and breakfast cereal.

"Uh-huh," she says. "It's so."

Across from us, Robert shakily struggles with his tomato plant, which seems to be falling over. The straighter the plant gets, the more crooked Robert becomes, his leg twisting under him, his arms straining.

"Do you need help?" I ask, worried he will fall.

"You're not strong enough to help," he tells me. "I can get it."

Mom watches him with great concentration. Finally, just when I think he's going to collapse onto the ground, he rights the plant and hobbles over to a bench to rest. Florence glides by, muttering, plucking up a leaf from the rosebush and batting at one of the tomatoes.

"Hey, wait," Robert says. "Come back here, I want to show you something."

I scoot even closer to Mom and show her another picture in the magazine, a cartoon of an octopus cooking pancakes. She laughs. "Silly," she says, and I feel a little swell of excitement that she has understood what she's looking at.

A plump, gray-and-white bunny, one of the outdoor pets, lumbers past, hops to the open door of the nursing home, puts in one paw, then hops away.

Mom does not see the bunny but notices the golden rose right beside her.

"That's a yellow rose. You used to grow roses," I say, remembering the childhood hours I spent weeding among the peace lilies, crimson glories, and American beauties in my mother's modest rose garden.

I have developed an odd sort of monologue for my times with Mom, a combination of reality orientation (Today is Friday, it's hot and sunny), memory boosting (Remember when you and Dad planted all those rosebushes?), positive reinforcement (You are such a great and wonderful woman), and stream of consciousness (Now here's a picture of Bill Cosby cooking chili, but you probably don't care about Bill Cosby; you probably wish there was a picture of Cary Grant). Talking to my mother brings with it a great sense of freedom. I have no worry about sentence structure, intellectual content, transitions and flow, or depth or relevance. It's especially fun when she appears to be at least mildly receptive, as she is today.

Dorothy wakes up from her nap, and I smile at her. She gets out of the chair and clasps her hands.

"It's you," she exclaims. "I haven't seen you in ages." She takes my hand and kisses it.

"I'm happy to see you," I tell her. She kisses my hand again. Mom stares at a picture of a coffeepot in the magazine, not noticing the lavish attention I am getting.

"My god, it's been four hundred dollars since I've seen you," Dorothy says effusively. She tries to sit next to me, but there isn't room. I pull over a chair, and she sits in it and promptly falls back to sleep.

I feel a little sad that my brief flurry of adoration, however delusional, has ended.

"The crack or sack," Mom says, staring at a page as though she's trying to read.

Florence bats the tomato plant as she passes again. The bunny hops over to rest under a shady bush.

A breeze floats strands of my mother's silvery hair across my face. I close my eyes and pretend we're on a beach together. Then I look at my watch and realize it's time to go.

"I'll see you on Saturday," I say, as if she can understand.

On my way out, I stop at the nurses' station. "Will someone help Mom back inside in a few minutes?" I ask. I feel a little pang of guilt as I ask; how sad that I cannot walk my mother back to her bedroom. How sad that after all these years of having her own home, she now has only one half of a room. And yet, how lucky we are to have found this place and these people.

The male aide is leaning against the desk. "Of course," he says. "I will help your mama."

I leave, feeling the imprint of my mother's shoulder against mine, the wet enthusiasm of Dorothy's kiss now a dry memory on my hand.

Remembering the Forgotten

I forget how many things you can forget.

My mother reminds me.

We are sitting at a restaurant, my mother, my father, and I, our Saturday tradition. Mom sits at the very edge of the booth, ignoring her food. Her silvery hair is shiny and soft; her fingernails have been painted a flirty pink. Despite the heat, she wears a pink sweatshirt adorned with an appliqué of a cornucopia and a pair of navy sweatpants. I feel my father's worry rising as he hands her yet another fork with a spear of chicken. She smiles and hands it back to him. The concept of eating has not clicked in. She has forgotten food, forks, and mealtimes. Those areas of her mind are blackened out, like the World War II blackouts she experienced in London.

"It takes her a while to get used to eating sometimes," I remind Dad.

He shakes his head, and I sense his frustration and his despair.

I try to cheer him up by sharing good news about my brother's job. But Dad, who ordinarily loves hearing anything about his son, is too involved with Mom and the strips of uneaten chicken to enjoy what I'm telling him.

One hour after the meal begins, Mom picks up a piece of chicken with her fingers and eats it. By then, Dad is ready to leave.

I stand in front of Mom, take her hands, and say, "Come up, let's go," in the cheerful voice that sometimes gets her attention. She looks at me and shrugs. I try again, the joy of Alzheimer's being that you get many, many tries and no one accuses you of being repetitive. On the fourth try, she stands. Dad and I help Mom walk out of the restaurant.

I feel the weight of her leaning against me. I feel how she wants to give in to her torpor. I wonder what would happen if my mother and I just sank down, right there on the sidewalk, in a melted heap, not talking, not moving, just leaning against each other. In a way, it would be a relief to join with her and forget that normal people have to keep moving until they reach their destination. Normal people cannot stop where they are and fall apart in a puddle of sorrow and weariness.

The sunlight pours down on us; the temperature is more than ninety degrees. I open the car door and pat the seat to remind Mom to sit. She stands there, wobbling. I hold her up and try to raise one of her legs, to get the sitting movement started. She says, "Oh, dear, oh honey," in a willowy wail, and I feel her weight heavy against me.

Dad goes around, gets into the backseat from the other side, and calls to her. Mom stands, immobile, moaning, the heat eating into her and into me. I try to pull Mom away from the car, walk her around, then start the seating process again—my usual routine. But she won't budge. I try to raise her knee, but she remains fixed and rigid, captured by whatever rhymes and visions wiggle through her brain.

My own brain is swirling. What should I do? Who can help me? How ridiculous not to be able to get my own mother into a car! What if Mom never moves, never gets in the car, what then?

I hold Mom's waist, pushing down again so she'll get the sitting idea. My shoulders are burning with heat, my arms exhausted from holding her up. I hear a baby crying and people walking in and out of the restaurant. All of these people can get into a car in less than a minute. What will they think of our tableau, the silver-haired woman in a sweatshirt and long pants, the brown-haired woman in a sleeveless top and slacks, standing as though under arrest against the inner car door?

Finally, Mom collapses and I catch her weight with my knee. It takes all my strength to pivot her and let her plop onto the edge of the car seat.

I wipe the sweat off my neck and kneel in the parking lot. After three tries, I get one of Mom's feet inside the car, then the other. A white shoestring dangles out of the door when I quickly shut it.

"Your mother's changing," Dad says as I drive back to the nursing home.

Mom's tilted against him in an awkward position, like a mannequin that hasn't been assembled properly.

"I think she's confused by anything unfamiliar right now," I say, while biting back my frustration.

"I sure don't want to go through this again," he says, and I hear the deep disappointment in his voice.

Our luncheon outings are acts of hopefulness. For Dad, the normal act of eating together in a restaurant means maybe Mom's mind could still return. Maybe, in the middle of a meal, she could turn to him and say, "Hi, Paul, I feel like we've been out of touch for a while. I feel like I've been on a strange and disturbing journey." Like Dad, I don't want to give up our rituals; I don't want to forget those simple, normal things.

"I think Mom needs a wheelchair to get to her room," I tell Dad.

Reluctantly, he agrees.

At the entrance to the nursing home, a long-haired, youngish man in a wheelchair sits smoking. He lives in the nursing home section, and I've seen him having wheelchair races in the parking lot with an even younger man who also lives there. I wonder at all he has forgotten: the sensation of feet pounding against asphalt, the feel of smooth loafers sliding along a wooden dance floor, the feeling of dirt between his toes. Dad goes to find a nurse and a wheelchair. I open the back door of the car, kneel on the ground, and take Mom's hands. She looks into space, then notices me and smiles.

"You're wonderful," she says. "It's wonderful, isn't it wonderful."

She sits there, a woman who has forgotten how to put her own good feet on the ground and rise up out of a car, a woman who has forgotten all the things that used to fuel her life. The woman who has forgotten everything says, "La la la," and laughs and reminds her daughter to enjoy what is happening right now.

"It's wonderful," Mom says again, swinging our hands.

"You're right," I say. If Mom were in her ordinary mind, I'd never be kneeling in the parking lot in front of her, holding her hands. She would worry about dirt on my slacks and what people might think. She would worry we were dawdling, being silly and unproductive. She would never giggle and smile at me in the innocent and delighted way she's doing right now.

For the first time today, I relax. Mom counts to seventeen. Dad and a nurse aide appear and we get Mom into the wheelchair. There are no footrests, so Mom scrapes her feet along the ground. The aide can barely push the chair, with Mom stopping the progress with her feet.

"Nice day, isn't it?" says the long-haired man who has forgotten what it's like to walk down the pavement. He taps out a fresh cigarette and smooths his breeze-ruffled ponytail.

I reach down and scoop up Mom's feet. She laughs. She hasn't forgotten that—how to laugh, how to smile, how to be silly and playful.

"Yes, it is a nice day," I answer as I inch forward, trying to keep my mother's feet just slightly off the ground.

The Glorious Movement

"You need a break," Ron tells me. He is trying to rub the tension out of my shoulders. I am so tired that I cannot argue with him. The responsibility of worrying over, staying connected with, and helping my parents is wearing me down. Squeezed in between work and other responsibilities, I spend hours each week with Mom and Dad. I am grateful they are near me, but I am also exhausted.

"A meditation retreat is just what you need," Ron advises. "Three days of silence and contemplation."

Normally, I am too restless to consider such an experience. But now, this seems like a relatively guilt-free chance to get away.

Before I go off to my retreat, I visit my mother. In the Alzheimer's unit, Mom is on her own sort of meditative retreat, complete with lots of sitting and walking practice.

Though it is an hour after lunch has been served, Mom sits alone in the dining room, a spoon in one hand, a green bean in the other.

"She dawdles over her food, but she gets it down," Ella, one of the nurse aides, reports. "We just let her sit there until she finishes. Why hurry her?"

I sit beside Mom, pat her back while she considers the lone green bean in her hand and the five beans clustered on her plate. I feel her calmness and try to still my tapping fingers, my bouncing knee. I am in a hurry to get in the car and drive to the retreat center so I can begin a period of silence, contemplation, and relaxation.

"When you go to lunch, focus only on your food," the retreat leader tells us the next day, after the morning meditation session. "Do not look at other people. Chew every bite mindfully. Put down your fork between bites. Try to keep your mind clear."

On this three-day silent retreat, we are practicing doing everything, from walking to eating, mindfully and with concentration.

During the first hours of the retreat, I felt restless and uncomfortable. But now I am relieved not to have to look at anyone, or smile or make any sort of small or large talk. The retreat is held at a Catholic monastery in a rural area. As we walk to the lunch area, the priests walk briskly past, their long, black robes flapping in the wind. I move behind two of them and overhear a conversation about updating the computer program. As I listen to arguments for various operating systems, I try to concentrate on my own operating system, the placing of the ball of my foot on the ground, the surrender of the heel, the movement of walking.

In the cafeteria line, I bow my head and hold my tray, like I am back in fourth grade. In grade school, the cafeteria line was a raucous place, the girls giggling and whispering, the boys showing off. This line is demure and silent. The cooks are large women from small towns. Before they come to work, they feed their men big farm breakfasts with ham, bacon, grits, biscuits, eggs, and strong coffee. They are puzzled by our silent group of pale people who want such weird and uninteresting vegetarian food.

"I'm making them some chocolate-chip cookies for dessert, just in case they're starving for something real to eat," the head cook had informed our retreat manager.

It's a good thing heads are lowered as the group of health-conscious organic-carrot juicers, flaxseed swallowers, vegan converts, tofu touters, and quinoa devotees go through the food line. Large aluminum bowls like my mother had in the 1950s swim with canned peaches (in, God forbid, heavy syrup). American cheese, sweet gherkins, and white bread grace the sandwich tray, while hopeful mounds of potato salad drenched with Miracle Whip (a much better choice than Hellman's in a holy place) complete the picnic. The salad bar, a special request that we paid extra for, is a wooden bowl with depressed iceberg lettuce, some grim cucumber slices, and some glossy-looking diced tomatoes.

One by one, we serve ourselves, and then sit down at long tables to eat. Each bite is an event, the slow movement of fork to mouth, the food deposited on the tongue, cradled in the mouth, and then slowly tasted as we begin chewing. I try to stay centered on the spiritual solemnity of this occasion. But out of the corner of my eye, I see the cook surveying us anxiously. She carries a tray with chocolate-chip cookies and sets it on a table next to brochures for other retreats. I take a bite of the canned fruit and hear the cookies calling me. I close my eyes and chew, willing the food to enter into me as a sacred fuel. One half-hour later, when my meager meal is mindfully consumed, I arise and force myself to walk slowly to the cookie tray. There are three cookies left.

By the last afternoon meditation, I am wishing I could go to my room, read a book, and plunder a bag of potato chips. My back hurts, my mind is swirling with ideas, and I am longing to break into a run and a shout. I stand still, calm myself, and walk slowly to the cafeteria. I keep my head lowered and try to erase the buzzing thoughts that arise at the sight of the peaches, drab lettuce, and mashed potatoes that came from a package.

As I bow my head over my plate, I think of my mother. She would be the star of this retreat, with her uncanny ability to hold a bite of mashed potato in her left hand and stare ahead, focused on a dot on the far wall.

"Take this practice home with you," the teacher tells us at the end of the retreat. "Try to stay connected with yourself and live in the present. Try not to rush back into everyday life."

It's my mother who brings me back into the present two days later, when I have already walked quickly, eaten breakfast in the car, and forgotten to get up early to meditate. I am saved from utter sloth and distraction by the practice of watching my mother.

I bring in lunch for both of us. I set up plates and serve her food. She does not recognize or acknowledge the food. I put a piece of shrimp on a fork and bring it to her mouth. She jerks away. I wait. She simply sits. I feel a panic rising. I have let go of wanting Mom to talk coherently, walk quickly, sit down easily, or toilet herself, but I want her to remember how to eat.

I hear the teacher's voice: "Things will always be there to interfere with and interrupt your practice. Try to be present with where you are."

I coach myself to simply be present, to enjoy my mother exactly as she is. Only after five minutes does she notice I am holding out a fork with something on it. She lets that something go into her mouth. She chews. She notices the plate. She sits. She stares. She nods off to sleep. She finds her hand, picks up a piece of shrimp and a bean sprout, and brings them to her mouth. She chews. The bean sprout drops into her lap. She picks up another shrimp, and sauce plops onto her shirt. Her hands are gleaming with food remnants. She falls asleep, she wakes, she stares, she eats, each act seeming to have the same importance.

I watch, knowing that someday she may not remember how to lift her hand to her mouth and eat. Someday she may just sit. I concentrate, in a way I could not at the retreat, on the glorious movement of my mother's hand to her mouth.

Digging

"I'd like to drive up and visit you, but I'm not sure I can stand to see Frances," a family friend says, her voice quiet.

"You can come visit me without seeing her," I say calmly.

Our friend is a brave woman and has weathered a lot in her life. But perhaps seeing Mom in such a depleted mental state is too much for her. Perhaps she wants to keep her image of my mother like a beautiful cameo, a memory she can still pull out and enjoy.

Walking into the Alzheimer's unit can change all that.

Because I live close to Mom and see her often, I am mostly used to her as she is. I have trained myself to walk up to my mother as though she is a partially excavated archeological site: Maybe today I'll find something to treasure.

When I was a kid, I would go to great lengths to get my mom's attention. I tugged at her skirt, plopped down right beside her, and leaned hard against her. I would loudly sing and twirl around.

Now I find myself taking much the same approach.

Today Mom is slumped over in a chair, looking just like the old ladies I remember being so scared of the first time I walked through a nursing home at age thirteen. Our neighborhood theater group was going to perform at the home, and we went over for an obligatory tour. As I walked beside my two best friends and behind the boy I had a crush on, I saw people who seemed like leftover foods forgotten on the plate—leaning, slumping, drooping, sleeping, drooling, fluttering, or staring, all in plain sight. That could never happen to me, I had vowed.

Now, years later, I am more humbly aware of how little I control my destiny.

Our friend would hate seeing Mom, slumped and lethargic, in the back row of the activities room, just outside the circle of other patients. Marci, the head of the unit, is facilitating a conversation, trying to engage all the patients. Mom seems oblivious. I bend down so I am right in front of Mom. Her eyes are glazed; she does not seem to notice me.

Marci notices me, waves, and smiles.

"We're talking about summertime," Marci tells me. "Now Elizabeth, what did you like about summertime when you were a kid?" Marci asks. She has the perfect voice for her audience, loud and friendly, firm and warm.

"Freedom," says Elizabeth. "We didn't work as much in summer."

"Mischief," says Claud, who is visiting his wife.

Everyone else is silent.

"Stan, how about you? Do you have some summer memories?"

Stan sits forward in his chair. His pushiness and energy are unusual here. He looks like a man who created his own business, who played poker with the guys, and liked Vegas. He looks like a man who drives a hard bargain.

"I have some memories, but I can't talk about them. I only have them at four o'clock." he says.

"I understand," Marci says and turns to Peggy.

I tap on Mom's arm. I stroke her shoulder. Just because I am a grown woman and my mother is deep into Alzheimer's doesn't mean I don't still want her attention. I say her name and wiggle my fingers in front of her. Finally, she sees me and laughs.

"Oh, you," she says.

I smile. I can imagine, if I wish, that she is really talking to me, her daughter. Or, I can just enjoy her smile, which, as always, is brilliant.

As Marci continues talking about summertime, I wonder what Mom's summertime memories might be. I'm pretty sure she rolled down a hill in Steubenville, Ohio, where she lived as a child. She might have watched her older sisters get dressed for dates. Did she ever go swimming? Did she play with friends? The answers are all part of what has been lost and buried. If Marci called on me, as my mom's spokeswoman, I wouldn't know how to answer.

And what was she doing in the summertime while I was growing up? In my early years, she was at home making Kool-Aid, visiting with neighbors, driving us to camp, or swimming. She turned on the garden hose so we could play in it. She dug in her purse for money, so we could buy Dreamsicles and Nutty Buddies from the ice cream man. She fanned herself and warned my brother and me we'd be sent to our rooms if we didn't stop fighting. She climbed up the pull-down steps into the sweltering attic, looking for old skirts, hats, and coats for our games of dress-up. She hung our clothes out to dry on the sagging wire lines that stretched across the backyard. She created a papier-mâché cow mask for our neighborhood theatrical productions and helped us make programs and flyers. She was the backdrop for every scene, a constant stage hand, and frequent director. Now I wonder: Did she like doing those things? Was she happy back in those days? Did she ever wish she were someplace else?

Marci reminisces about her own childhood, and the conversation continues around the circle. Meanwhile, Mom drifts away from me. I wave my fingers, make a face, show her a photograph of my daughter as a baby, and shake the shiny red Mardi Gras bead necklace I carry with me on my visits. Sometimes she likes the shine of the beads. Sometimes she's drawn to the baby pictures. Today, she just laughs and says, "It's silly."

"I don't know if I can stand it, seeing her like that," our friend had told me. I heard the break in her voice—she who had already lost so much.

"Just come see me," I say. "If you don't want to see Mom, it's all right. Really, it's all right."

Yet part of me wants our friend to love the shards that are left, the sudden gleam of recognition, like treasure found. Nothing is on the surface these days, no signs of the exalted civilization that once inhabited my mother. She can no longer describe her experiences in the Shakespeare Club, where she and her friends read and discussed all of the Bard's works. Though a couple of her original oil paintings hang in the nursing home, she cannot point to them with shy pride. She no longer remembers her stories of serving in Iceland and England during World War II. Those were the last of her stories, and at the time I thought I'd always be able to hear her tell them. Now I am kneeling on the dirt, with small brushes. I am carefully searching for remnants of the beauty that once was—a sentence fragment, a scrap of memory, a spark of delight at a long-loved picture, a bite of a favorite candy bar.

An hour can go by and there is simply no sign of life. Then my mother says, "There's a pie." (And there is a piece of pie nearby.) I'd love for our friend to experience that swell of excitement, that joyous cry, the hallelujah of hope, before dust and time take over and everything is hidden once again.

IV.
Fight and Surrender:
2002–2003

Radio Ways

One of my earliest memories of Dad was in Wynne, Arkansas, when Dad worked the night shift at the radio station. One night, when I couldn't sleep, Mom took me and my baby brother up to see where Dad worked. The building had a large inner atrium, and the radio station had a glassed-in studio on the second floor. When we entered the building, I looked up and saw my dad, high above me, like God. I heard his voice, mellow and deep, like God's, and heard him say my name over the air, dedicating a song to me and to my brother.

Dad fell in love with radio in his early twenties when he was flunking out as a medical student.

In his first radio job, he worked from 6:00 a.m. until 2:00 p.m. for station WLNH in Laconia, New Hampshire. He received fifteen bucks a week and his duties included reading the news, selecting the music (mostly easy listening), acting as disk jockey, reporting sports, and sweeping up before each shift. He also monitored the network programming that came in on his shift.

After the war, he worked as program director at WKBR in Manchester, New Hampshire. Initially, Dad worked from 6:00 a.m. to noon (he still swept up before each shift and still did news, sports, music, DJ-ing, and remotes). After his shift on the radio, he got into his 1929 Studebaker and drove to Rockingham Race Track, where he worked at the ten-dollar window for thoroughbred racing.

Here's what my father wrote to Frances about radio work: "It's interesting enough, though far less glamorous than the average person believes. It becomes hard work day after day to fool the public into believing you're happy all the time."

Years later, as Mom moved more deeply into Alzheimer's, Dad replayed his radio training. He tried to fool the nurse aides, the kitchen staff, the other families, and my brother and me into thinking he was happy, or at least coping. But we knew him too well. We could see and feel the pain and anguish underneath his brittle smile. We could see the hard, hard work of all he was going through.

The Birthday Girl

"How would your mother like to celebrate her birthday?" Dad asks me over dinner one evening. We are seated in a family restaurant, eating cherry pie and drinking decaf coffee.

I take a bite of the sticky-sweet pie and think about Mom, sitting in front of the TV in the Alzheimer's unit, one minute slumped in her chair like a doll without stuffing, another moment smiling and laughing at whatever is right in front of her. There is no way of knowing which persona would be present on her birthday. There is no promise of even a smile or a look of recognition on the momentous occasion of her eighty-seventh year.

"I think this birthday celebration is for you and me," I say. "I think we are honoring Mom's long and wonderful life. Mom may not even know it's her birthday."

"What about gifts?" Dad's voice sounds tired and strained.

"I don't think Mom needs gifts," I say.

A gift is simply an addition to the photographs, knickknacks, and magazines that collect in the Alzheimer's unit. Mom might pick up a photo in Judy's room and drop it off on Stan's bed. Sally Jo might pick up the doll that Fay's daughter had laid carefully on the bedside just the night before and deliver it to the cleaning cart.

"What about cake?" Dad asks.

"Yes, cake would be great."

Dad smiles just a little. I see how hard this birthday is for him—his beloved wife there in the flesh, yet not there in the mind.

"Maybe we should just forget it," Dad says, sadness seeping through his voice.

"No. You and I need to celebrate," I say.

I ask Ron to go with me to the party. We need lots of energy and hopefulness to get through this birthday.

When we arrive, Mom is sitting at the lunch table, as always the last one to finish her meal. She has on lipstick and blush. Her hair is clean and brushed. Her manicured fingers are caked with food. Dad sits beside her, a discouraged expression on his face.

"Hi, Mom." I wave in a silly exaggerated way, and Mom laughs.

"Aren't you wonderful," she says, taking Ron's hand and then mine.

"She didn't even acknowledge me," Dad says.

Mom laughs and looks down at her lap.

"Where's the cake?" I ask, and Dad unveils a magnificent sheet cake with purple writing and white icing.

"Where are the people?" Ron asks.

"Scattered everywhere." Dad waves his hand tiredly.

Ron springs into action, walking around and encouraging people to come into the dining room. George, the nurse in charge, hands me paper plates, napkins, and a knife to cut the cake. I slice big, gooey pieces. Propelled by Ron's enthusiasm, people drift in and settle around the tables. George pours orange drinks. I serve Mom first, a piece of cake with a flower, as befits a birthday girl. Mom picks up the cake and holds it upside down in her hand, icing against her palm. I try to stick a plate under the cake, but she moves her hand protectively away.

"Want me to cut it into bites for you, Mom?"

She doesn't answer; just bends and takes a bite of cake, crumbs clinging to her face and falling onto her white slacks.

We pass cake and drinks to each patient. A nurse aide arrives with Dixie cups of vanilla ice cream. People murmur over the cake and ice cream. Stan reaches over and takes Fay's cake. Fay takes Edna's cake. We serve Edna another piece. Mom holds her cake, eating it little by little.

"This reminds me of you on your second birthday," Dad tells me as I mop up a spilled drink. "You grabbed onto a slice of cake and would not let go. Your mother said, 'Why not? It's one day a year. Let her eat the way she wants to.'"

I smile at Dad and see him relax a little. The tension lifts from his face and he looks at my mom with affection and delight. I think about my kids and the way I had delighted over them getting messy with their early birthday cakes. I sometimes wish I could still dive into a birthday cake with that same sense of joy and abandon, but manners always get in the way.

"Every year is a new beginning, a chance to discover a new part of yourself," I once read in a spiritual text.

What would this year, this mysterious golden crone's eighty-seventh year, bring to my mother, I wonder, as I watch her lower her head to her palm and take a nip of frosting. Her fingernails are filled with icing, her cheeks blushed with white sugar. She looks at her messy hands and laughs.

Dad laughs too. "That's right, Frannie, have fun with this," he says.

"Your mother is one wonderful woman," says George, pouring another drink. "And your father is one wonderful man."

Mom laughs at the peaks of frosting on her hand. If you ask her, "What is this day?" she can't answer you. If you ask her, "Where are you and how old are you and who are these people sitting around you, paying such close attention to you?" she can't say.

She can't even make a birthday wish or blow out her candles.

But she can lower her face to the glob of celebration nestled right in her own palm and she can raise her face and laugh.

"Happy birthday, Mom," I say, kissing her messy cheek and tasting its sweetness.

The Woman She Was

My friend Karen gives me a gift: She says, "Tell me about your mother."

We are sitting in a quiet café in midafternoon, and I let the question sink in.

When friends occasionally ask me, "How is your mother doing?" I have different answers, depending on the situation. If we are in one of those conversations that are like confetti in brisk wind, I say, "She's okay."

If we are sitting across from each other and my friend is looking right at me, I answer, "She's pretty deep into Alzheimer's."

"Does she recognize you?" she might ask.

"No, but she may recognize I am a person she likes," I answer.

That usually ends that conversation.

But "Tell me about your mother" is an invitation I don't usually get.

"What would you like to know?" I ask.

She stirs her iced mocha. "Whatever you want to tell me," she says softly. "I would like to know about her life and her interests."

Since my mother has been in the nursing home with Alzheimer's, I have seldom talked about the person she used to be. Occasionally my father and I reminisce about family vacations and outings. I sometimes ask Dad questions about our growing-up days and the early days of their courtship. But I rarely think about the woman I knew all my life, the mother, grandmother, artist, gardener, compassionate friend, avid reader, bird-watcher, early-morning walker, lemon-meringue pie baker. That woman is gone, and I have spent a lot of energy learning how to know and appreciate the woman who now commandeers her body.

As I consider what I want to tell Karen, I remember visiting my mom's best friend, Bel, in California when I was a teenager. Bel, who was spunky and adventurous in a way that seemed so different from my conservative mother, drove me from Berkeley to the small resort where I would work as a chambermaid for the summer.

"Do you know how I met your mom?" she asked me as we drove down the winding roads, past fragrant stands of eucalyptus trees.

"In Iceland, during World War II," I said. I had heard stories of the two of them taking a break from their work in the hospital by skiing, then stopping for a soak in a hot spring.

"No, we met earlier in Chicago. We were both nurses working the twelve-hour night shift. The hospital had a room with a couple of bunk beds so we could rest on breaks. One night I walked in there and heard the most heartbreaking sobbing. It was Frances, crying her eyes out. I asked her what was wrong and she said, 'Nothing.'"

I smiled. That sounded like Mom, never wanting to admit anything was wrong.

"Then I asked her again and she sobbed that her husband Sam had died six months ago from pneumonia. She was so sad, she didn't know if she could go on. A bunch of other nurses and I were going to Florida for a short vacation, and I persuaded your mother to join us. But as it turned out, we never went; a week later I decided to join the army and I encouraged her to come along. We've been best friends ever since."

When I heard this story at the age of seventeen, I was too young to fathom my mother's grief and despair. By the time I told Karen the story, I had some sense of what my mother must have gone through.

"Your mom was really brave, to serve in the army during wartime," Karen says.

I feel a little swell of pride. Mom's tales of traveling in the darkest night on the troop ship, with bombs falling nearby, were so familiar that I had never considered her bravery.

Now I tell Karen how my father, encouraged by Bel's husband, wrote Mom a letter, telling her he was ready to marry a nice Jewish girl. Was she interested? Was she available?

After some correspondence, Mom surprised herself by agreeing to meet him in Chicago. At the end of the week, my father asked her to marry him. She considered the offer for three weeks and accepted. Their whirlwind romance was fueled by practicality.

"What a great story," Karen says. "Your mother must be an amazing woman."

Sparked by Karen's interest, I let myself feel my love for my mother as she used to be. I am in tears by the time our conversation ends.

"Thank you for asking me about my mother," I say to Karen.

"Your stories make me want to call my own mom and hear her stories again."

As I drive home, I think of more "Mom" stories to share with my children and my brother. I see myself, along with my brother and father, as the carrier of my mother's sacred legacy. I imagine myself tenderly fanning the embers, adding dry leaves and crumpled paper, creating a blaze with each memory. I realize I don't have to give up Mom's old self: I can be her historian and her scribe, carrying her stories with me and making sure they live on.

The Great-Grandmother's Diaper

"You'll need this for your outing," the nurse says.

The large disposable diaper rustles as I try to figure out where and how to carry it. Can I roll it up and stuff it in my pocket, or fold it neatly enough to slide into my purse? And how exactly does the diaper work?

"It works just like a regular diaper," the nurse tells me, handing me a plastic sack.

I want to inform her that a regular diaper is for a helpless, adorable, growing, squirming baby, whereas this diaper is slated for my mother. Though I have taken Mom on many short outings, I have never had to deal with her diaper. Today, she is going to be with me all afternoon. I need to be prepared.

"She may get through the afternoon fine without it," the nurse says, patting my shoulder. "I'll be here all day. If you have any questions or need anything, just call me."

I said similar words to my daughters' babysitters, years ago. I laid out diapers, formula, baby food, extra towels, and baby blankets. I had given them my phone number, my sister-in-law's phone number, my neighbor's phone number, my best friend's phone number, and, of course, a list of emergency numbers.

Right now, this simple trip across town with a woman I've known and loved all my life seems daunting. I feel like I am on an outing with a complete stranger. And in a sense, I am.

"Come on, Fran, you're going with your daughter," the nurse says. Mom sits in a nearby chair, rocking back and forth, fiercely rubbing the top of her head, her face in a grimace.

I imagine a television announcer saying, "This is your mother," and flashing to a photo of a smiling, waving Fran, only seven years ago. "This is your mother on Alzheimer's," the announcer then says, and indeed, here she is, right in front of me.

The nurse holds out her hand and Mom stops rocking. She looks at the nurse and smiles.

"All right," she says. "All right."

As the nurse walks her over to me, Mom smiles.

"We're going to my house, Mom. You're going to meet your great-granddaughter."

"Whatever," Mom says cheerfully.

My niece is visiting from Colorado with her year-old daughter, Sofia, my parents' first great-grandchild. My father is elated! What an accomplishment, what a thrill, what a deep blessing to see this magical new generation. He has told Mom all about Sofia, has shown her pictures and tried his best to prepare her for the visit.

But in her current state of disconnection, Mom doesn't require prep time. She is strictly a woman of the present.

I wonder what my tall, beautiful niece, Helen, thinks when she sees me leading her doddering grandmother into the house, a grandmother who just a few years ago read novels, baked butterscotch brownies, walked miles, and listened attentively to her grandchildren. I wonder what sense of loss, shock, or outrage courses through her. But Helen is above all a gracious and kind woman, and instantly gives Mom a gentle, loving hug.

"Hello, Nana," she says, calling Mom by her grandmotherly name. "It's Helen."

"Helen," Mom says, rolling the word over her tongue as if it were coated with chocolate. "You're so pretty."

"And Nana, this is Sofia." Helen points to her baby, who sits happily on the floor, playing with an assortment of toys.

My father sits on the sofa, watching Sofia with a look of rapture. The adoration stays in his eyes as he rises to hug Mom and guide her to the sofa. They sit side by side, my father pointing out the baby to Mom.

Then Sofia stands up on her wavering, wobbling new legs and walks over to my mother. She places her hands on Mom's knees, moving back and forth. A bubble of drool blooms on her lips. She smiles sweetly.

"Da!" she reports.

"Ah, ah baby," my mother says, beaming, looking right at Sofia. "What a pretty baby."

Sofia plops down, then crawls over to grab a toy car. Gripping the car, she toddles over to Mom and presents her with the toy. Mom pats the baby's hand. My father watches, smiling. Helen watches, smiling. I watch, entranced.

"This is your great-granddaughter, Frannie," Dad says. He had been sure that if Mom ever got to see this child, something magical would happen. He had hoped that this baby would boost Mom into remembering the rest of her family—Helen, Dan, me—but he will settle for Mom simply enjoying the baby.

I put down the sack that contains the adult diaper, sit down beside my niece, and watch Mom and the baby.

How does Sofia know to walk over to my mother? How does she sense that Mom needs her delightful charm?

For one hour, Sofia tirelessly toddles back and forth between her toys and her great-grandmother. For one hour, Mom watches every move that delicious child makes. Then Sofia picks up her stuffed turtle, rubs her eyes, and sticks out her lip.

"She's tired," Helen says, rising to pick up her daughter. "She's wet and she's ready for her nap. Say goodnight to Nana, Sofia." Sofia puts her head on Helen's shoulders and closes her eyes.

While Sofia naps and Helen reads, I serve my parents cookies and coffee. Dad and I talk about the baby. We discuss every movement, every smile, every interaction with Mom. Then I notice Mom is nodding, her cookie crumbling on the leg of her slacks, her coffee cup wavering in her hand. I rescue the food and wonder if Mom is wet. But I can't bear the idea of easing my hand under the top of Mom's diaper to find out.

What kind of a daughter leaves her mother wearing the same diaper for four hours? A wet diaper can cause rash. The wet might feel oppressive and uncomfortable against Mom's skin. Still, I cannot walk over to the plastic sack and take out the white rectangle of protective paper. I cannot take my mother's hands and guide her into the bathroom. I am not ready to take another step away from being her daughter, toward being her caretaker.

An hour later, I drive my sleepy mother back to the nursing home and walk her to the Alzheimer's unit.

"How did she do?" the nurse asks.

"Great. The baby played with her and she loved it."

Then the nurse notices the sack with the diaper, which I am gripping in my right hand.

"I can't believe I'm so intimidated by a diaper," I tell her. "I just couldn't deal with it."

"Most families feel that way," the nurse says calmly, leading Mom to the bathroom.

I hurry back home. Perhaps Sofia will be up from her nap. Perhaps I will sit on the floor and play with her, holding nothing in my mind but her charming curiosity and the sudden surprise of her smile.

And perhaps when she gets wet, I will get up willingly and, with great calm and confidence, change her diaper.

Wanted: Another Mother

"Okay, Mom, I've had enough," I say, standing up and folding my arms across my chest. "Really, if you don't start paying more attention to me, I'm going to have to do something drastic. I'm going to have to find another mother. Mom, are you listening? Mom?"

Mom is definitely not listening, which is, of course, part of the problem.

I walk out of the Alzheimer's unit, my hands clenched, my jaw tight. I knew this would happen. I understand the progression of the disease. What I didn't understand is how much I would miss having a mother.

I get into the car, feeling like a small child having a big fit. I realize if I want any semblance of the sort of mother figure I am used to, I will have to go out and find her. I am not going to abandon my own mother; I just want to supplement her.

I envision my personal ad:

MAD Desires OM for LTR
Middle-Aged Daughter Desires Other
Mother for Long-Term Relationship.
Seeking bright, opinionated, literate,
compassionate older woman.
Must be a good listener. A propensity for sweets preferred.

I know there are wonderful adoption programs for older children who need good homes. Is there a venue for midlife women who are either orphaned or feel motherless? Perhaps some entrepreneurial Internet expert can create *Match.mom*. Wouldn't some lonely elder goddess-crone enjoy having me as her surrogate child?

At the grocery store, I study the women as I push my cart down the aisles. What kind of mother do I want? Do I want a mother in the proper age range, or will a loving, motherly woman my own age or slightly older do? Is body type an issue? My own mother is slender, but perhaps this time I want a plus-size mom. And what of personality? My mother was a great listener, always eager to hear another person's issues and thoughts. Is that a requirement? Mom also had a lot of rules and opinions. Is a woman who likes to be in control a necessity?

For the next few weeks, as I go to meetings, do errands, and attend gatherings, I find myself gazing at older women and wondering, "Would you like to be my other mother?"

Right away, I find several excellent candidates. One friend's mom, in her eighties, is an avid volunteer, card player, and reader. She is kind and thoughtful and also opinionated in a way similar to my mom.

Another friend, who spent her seventy-fifth birthday camping in the Sahara, would make an adventuresome and outgoing mother. Yet another friend, only in her mid-sixties, has warmth and compassion, and a gift for baking. I imagine what a cozy, comforting mom she would make.

I decide to treat the other-mother-selection process like I am filling a high-powered job. I create an interview form, featuring questions such as:

- What makes a good mother–daughter relationship?
- How many daughters do you currently have? (I didn't want too much competition.)
- What is your definition of success?
- What do you like to read?
- What kinds of topics do you like to talk about?
- What special qualities do you have to offer as my other mother?

I imagine inviting each potential mother figure to lunch, my questions at the ready. I imagine they all have excellent listening skills, compassion, wit, and appropriate interest in arts and literature. They each answer easily, forthrightly, with focus and thoughtfulness. They are nicely dressed, health-conscious without being fanatical, and easy to be around.

I would have no problem claiming any one of them as one of my most important relatives.

"How's the search for your new mother coming?" a friend asks. Her own mother died some years ago, and she is watching me closely, in case my idea turns out to be a good one.

"I have three amazing candidates, but something's missing. I can't figure out what," I tell her.

Meanwhile, I visit my real mom. I note the contrast: Instead of meeting a well-groomed, articulate woman at a nice restaurant, I punch a red button and enter the locked Alzheimer's ward.

Louise, a new patient, walks toward me.

"Hello," I say as she rushes up.

"Oh hello, I'm so happy to see you. I don't know what I'm supposed to be doing," she says. Her cheeks glow with the flush of new roses. Her pink sweater is clean and properly buttoned. *Is this my other mother?* I wonder briefly.

She walks with me as I look around for Mom.

She is in her room, asleep, angled across the bed with her feet on the ground. I watch her for a while, and then I tap her leg. She opens her eyes. I wave at her. She smiles. I wave harder.

She laughs. The anxiety that sometimes grips her, causing her to rub her hands against her head or to yank at her clothes, has temporarily melted away. She is simply a beautiful, silver-haired woman. I keep silent and look into Mom's eyes. She looks into my eyes. The air is pure and sweet between us. There is no misunderstanding, no lost thoughts, no forced or garbled sentences. We are two creatures gazing at each other with openness and compassion. I hear the nurse aides going about their work, the patients walking down the corridor. I hear the large cart that carries the lunch dishes rumbling down the hallway. But those sounds are background music—I am only connected with my mother.

As I look into her eyes, I wonder: *What makes us walk away from our mothers and then run back? What makes us pretend we are not our mothers—that we have nothing in common with these women? What lets us imagine we are going to be so much stronger, smarter, and happier than they were?* When I was younger, I spent a lot of time separating myself from my mother. Now, I want to be closer.

I sink into my mother's face like she is a meditation. We smile at each other for a half-hour, something we have never done before, something that would be too intense, too personal in our earlier, rational life together.

Then her eyes gently flutter shut. I feel like I've been on a mystical retreat. I feel a rich sense of renewal and hope.

As I watch my mother fall into slumber, I realize I don't really want another mother. I like the softer, less controlled persona of this mother. I like her silly noises and ready laughter. I like the fact that she doesn't know who I am, but smiles at me anyway. I am growing comfortable with her new, unorthodox style of motherhood.

Mom's eyes are closed, her hands resting by her sides. I kneel on the floor and rest my head against her legs. I feel her warmth and the sureness of her breathing. Then I feel her hand on my head, tugging playfully at my curls, just like she used to do when I was a little girl. I smile, close my eyes, and rest.

The Answer Is Tom Cruise

"I think Tom Cruise is the answer," my dad says.

We are sitting in my mom's room in the Alzheimer's unit, Dad and I perched on the bed, Mom in a chair, bent over a photo album.

Was it only last month that she actually looked at the pictures, as if she might recognize them? Now, even with all our pointing and exaggerated enthusiasm, she barely notices the pictures underneath the plastic covering. She does notice the plastic covering and picks at a corner of it.

"Tom Cruise?" I ask. "Tom Cruise is the answer to what?"

Dad nods sagely and tells me this story.

My parents were celebrating their forty-something anniversary in one of Memphis's older and finer restaurants. They were seated at a quiet corner table, when a craning of heads and an increase in conversations prompted them to look around, and they spotted a handsome man striding through the restaurant. He seemed to have an entourage surrounding him, but he stopped to shake hands and sign napkins. Then he smiled, waved to the restaurant at large, and let himself be ushered into a private room.

"That Tom Cruise is one handsome man," Mom said as she and Dad settled back into their meal.

Dad looked up. He and Mom often discussed movies, but he had never heard her speak so definitively about a man's good looks.

"Shall I try to get him to come over and talk with us?" he asked. He was already planning just how he would make the approach—a private conversation with the waiter, who was already charmed by the length of their marriage. That conversation would lead to a more conspiratorial tête-à-tête with the aloof maître d' with occasional references to my mother, looking beautifully silver-haired and angelic as she nibbled on her salmon béarnaise.

"Oh, no," Mom said. "I don't want to talk to him. I just want to look at him."

Now, fifteen years after the almost-encounter with Tom Cruise, my dad is considering Mr. Cruise as one in a series of possible saviors—people, places, or events that can release my mother from her Alzheimer's prison and liberate her back into the woman she used to be.

"I believe when your mother sees Tom Cruise on the screen, she will know who he is and remember that evening we saw him," Dad tells me as we watch Mom get up to fold and refold a pillowcase. She pulls the blue, ribbed bedspread half up on the other bed, then sits down, then stands up, then pulls on the bedspread again.

"Do you want this?" she asks me, with a tone of exasperation in her voice.

"No, I don't need it. You can leave it right there."

Mom puts her hands on her hips, then leans down to pick up a piece of lint from the floor.

"Mom doesn't even know who I am half the time," I tell my father. "I am going to be very upset if she recognizes Tom Cruise. Plus, he could look different on the movie screen."

"I think she will recognize him," Dad says.

Dad tells me his plan: He envisions making a preliminary phone call to the manager at a nearby theater. "I am an older man. I am bringing my wife to the movies. But she's easily distracted and may not stay long. If she has to leave early, I'd like to arrange in advance for a refund." That way, if the movie is a failure, at least it will not cost too much.

The last time my mom went to the movies, she bolted out of the theater just after the opening credits and strode off into another theater in the multiplex. I ran after her and followed her inside, where she spent several minutes fiddling with the stuffing that was oozing out of the upholstered seats. Then she left that theater. She and I walked up and down the corridors, eating popcorn and Junior Mints, while Dad finished watching his movie.

"I don't think Mom can sit still even while she's waiting for the movie to start," I say to Dad. "I don't think she'll notice the screen. She doesn't even focus on the television when it's on."

"Perhaps we just haven't found the right movie. I believe that when she sees Tom Cruise, she'll remember almost meeting him. She'll sit and watch the movie."

Meanwhile, Mom sits on the bedspread and reaches under her orange stretch pants to explore the top of her adult diaper. Then she tugs again at the spread.

"What the heck is this?" she says. "It's candled, you bums."

I watch my Dad.

He explains to Mom it's a bedspread. He reminds Mom of the bedspread they had years ago, a beautiful ivory coverlet that my grandmother had crocheted.

My mom sits still while he talks, then continues her yanking. "You old so-and-so's," she says.

"I'm going to get a newspaper to see what the movie times are," Dad tells me. "Will you stay here with your mother?"

I watch my dad walk out of the room.

The head nurse will find him a paper. Maybe she will raise her eyebrows when she hears his plan. Maybe she will just nod and smile. She is used to my father's ideas and schemes.

"Your father is often unrealistic," she once told me.

"I know," I said. "I like that about him."

"Me too," she said.

Like me, she secretly wants one of his schemes to work.

He comes back with the paper.

"The movie is on at that little theater, the one just a few miles away. I think this could work. Right, Frannie?" he asks, raising his voice to get Mom's attention.

She looks up from opening a drawer and turns to my father as if he is a sudden full moon.

"Right," she says.

"Maybe you should walk in late, after the movie has started, so Tom might already be on the screen," I say, a spot of hope rattling around in me.

"Yes," Dad agrees. "That's a good idea. I'll bring a flashlight and guide us to our seats."

"Do you want me to come with you?" I ask.

"No, I think your mother and I need to do this together. We'll be fine, won't we, Frannie?"

"Whatever," Mom says, grabbing a fistful of her shirt.

Later that night, I get a call from Dad.

"Well?" I ask, hoping that something miraculous happened.

"Tom was on the screen when we walked in and I think she smiled. But I'm not sure she recognized him, with the makeup and different hair and such. And she didn't seem to understand how to sit down in the seats, so we left."

"Did you get your money back?"

"We got all our money back," Dad tells me proudly. "You know, I think you were right. She needs to see Tom Cruise in person. I'm going to call a promoter I know in Memphis and see if he can give me a lead."

I smile as I listen to Dad's latest plan. He has energy and a sense of hope in his voice that I haven't heard in months. I guess Tom Cruise is an answer, if not for my mother, at least for my dad.

A Doll of Her Own

That afternoon, while my mother is walking down the left-hand side of the corridor in the Alzheimer's unit, tapping one hand on the handrail and pressing the other palm on her forehead, she sees a baby doll lying on the floor. Mom's adult diaper rustles as she bends down, picks the baby doll up, smooths its curly hair, and carries it with her to the dining room. There she settles in a chair and rocks the doll, talking and singing to it.

"Your mom's fallen in love with a baby doll," Leticia, the nurse aide, says when I visit. "I've never seen anything quite like it."

Mom is sitting at the table in the small dining room, her head bent over as if she's fallen asleep on a long journey. I touch her shoulder once, twice, and on the third time she straightens, notices me, and smiles.

I sit beside her and spread out some photographs I have brought, pictures of people she used to know and now doesn't. She is staring vacantly at a photo of her granddaughters when Leticia brings over the baby doll.

"Here you go, Frances," Leticia says.

Mom lights up, holds out her arms, and begins talking. "You're cute. You're so pretty. You're a good boy. You're a good girl."

I look on in amazement. I haven't seen Mom so animated in weeks. Yet I feel a momentary pang: I had yearned to be the one who jolted her into vivacity. I watch her carefully. Was this what it was like when I was little? Did Mom's face grow bright and happy, and did she sit around and say sweet nonsense to me?

Three ladies congregate nearby, each of them watching the baby. Freda says, "She's sweet." Ethel just stares. Mary hits her fist against the wall and walks on.

Bill comes racing into the room. He wears his usual red cardigan, with one hole at the left elbow and a smear of food near the right pocket; his silver hair is neatly slicked back. He sits down as though he has only minutes to spare.

"Do you want to come into the rodum-dodum?" Mom asks the baby. She is talking in the high-pitched, singsong voice she used to reserve for little children. I realize I have never seen my mother holding a baby doll.

"You are such a good baby. I love you, yes sir," Mom says. Then she looks at me, as if I've suddenly come into the room.

"I like your outfit," she says. "That's a good outfit." I sit up straighter. I am always surprised and pleased when such a cogent remark tumbles out.

Mom takes one of the photographs I brought and shows it to the baby.

"Do you know who that is?" she asks, sounding much like I did a year or so ago, when I believed that seeing her family's pictures over and over again would help restore Mom's memory.

I listen as Mom continues her conversation with the baby. Maybe the ease of having someone who doesn't talk back, who doesn't hope you will complete a sentence, who doesn't care if the words are missing or not right, maybe that freedom lets Mom flow with her speech.

"I think Mom needs her own baby doll," I mention to Leticia as I leave.

"That doll sure gets her juices going," Leticia says.

The last time I shopped for dolls, my daughter Sarah was seven years old and in need of a Barbie. Buying my mother a baby doll seems like a life moment.

At the toy store, the baby dolls are all full of activities. One laughs when you press her belly. One has a musical bottle. Others take your picture with a camera or sing to you in Spanish. One baby knows four cheers. Not one of them is large enough, quiet enough, babylike enough.

I wonder if my mother had to search when she bought me my favorite doll, a present for my sixth birthday. My friends all got dolls that talked or moved that year. My doll, Sally, just listened. Sally had a calm presence that I adored all during my doll-playing years. I never really took to any other dolls, even the talking doll who appeared the next birthday; she was too glamorous, too sophisticated for me.

I want to find a doll for my mother like she had found for me, so many years ago. A doll without skills or frills that fits into your arms and listens.

I search the aisles for a quiet doll without too many accomplishments. Finally I find a soft, rosy-cheeked baby, a good size to cradle, who boasts only an open mouth for a pacifier or bottle.

"Some little girl is going to really enjoy this doll," the cashier says as I pay.

I smile as I envision that eighty-seven-year-old little girl who is my mother.

Back in the car, I feel a flutter of nervousness, like I had felt as a kid when I bought my mom presents. Will she like it; will she really like it? Will her face light up, or will she just ignore it?

Mom sits in a chair in the TV room, eating strawberry ice cream out of a round cardboard container. I know better than to compete with ice cream, so I wait until she has eaten the last smidgen.

Then I sit down beside her and put my hand on her shoulder. She looks at me, her eyes vacant and lost.

"Hi, Mom," I say. She stares at me, and then she sees the baby doll.

"You're here," she says, her eyes widening. "My little girl is here."

She holds out her arms and I hand her the baby.

"Bo bo bupe, tootle ootle, oop. I have my little girl," she croons.

She smiles at me; she smiles at the doll. Does she know I'm her real little girl, or is she imagining the doll as her child? At this moment, as I watch my mother come to life and praise her baby, it simply doesn't matter.

All That Glitters

For a couple of years, my mother's clothes have been crammed into three suitcases and stored in my basement. The pearl buttons, wire hooks, and smooth zippers of her good skirts, blouses, and dresses have given way to soft pullovers, expandable waists, sweatshirts, and sweatpants. About once a week I think about opening the suitcases, which my father packed, to see what is inside. Then something inside me tightens, and I end up doing nothing.

But last week, my daughter needed luggage for a trip, and Mom's suitcase with rolling wheels was perfect for her. I made myself go down the basement stairs. I squatted beside the case and glared at it. I had finally gotten used to seeing my mom in stained, appliquéd sweatshirts and baggy sweatpants. I did not want to be reminded of her more sophisticated days.

Finally, I unzipped the case. Inside was a jumble of old pajamas, slips, belts, and a few scarves. I trailed my hand through the soft pajamas and felt a pinch of sadness as I lifted out the sea-green scarf Mom had always worn with her black linen sheath. The scarf had a faint aroma of powder, and I imagined Mom at one the many parties she and my father threw or attended, holding a glass of chardonnay, the silken curves of color draped "just so" around her shoulders.

Then I caught a glimpse of black and a sparkle of silver. I pushed aside the rayon pink PJs and lifted out a glittery, black, long-sleeved top. My mother had bought this elegant piece for full price at an exclusive Memphis shop to celebrate one of her wedding anniversaries. I remembered a smiling photo of her and Dad, their heads together, the glittery top shining against Dad's dark suit.

I fingered the fabric, remembering how my mother loved its exuberant sparkle. This would fit me. *I could actually wear this sometime,* I thought.

The top and the pajamas smelled deeply of mildew, so I scooped them up, added them to my pile of dirty clothes, and began the laundry.

A couple of hours later, I reached into the dryer to take out the clean clothes. I pulled out a towel and noticed tiny sparkles dotting it. My black turtleneck and my jeans were similarly adorned. A purple shirt glistened with miniscule silver dots. My mother's glittery shirt had distributed its wealth, and the whole load of laundry was shining.

I'll have to wash everything again, I thought. But I didn't have time, so I carried the folded clothes upstairs and forgot about the sparkles.

Two days later, I was getting ready for an important meeting. I took a bath, toweled off, and dressed in slacks and a black turtleneck. When I went into the bathroom to brush my hair, I noticed my face looked like I was preparing for a New Year's Eve celebration—I had little specks of glitter on my cheeks and forehead. My top also was spattered with glitter. I rubbed at the glitter on my face—a few dots fell onto my slacks. I was running late, and I decided no one would notice my extra shine.

As I drove to the meeting, I remembered my mother standing before her mirror, wearing her satin dress, putting on her red lipstick and her clip-on rhinestone earrings. She sprayed on Chanel No. 5 and fastened on a matching rhinestone necklace. She was going to a party with my father, and she looked glamorous and glittery. I sat on her bed and watched her transformation from sensible, plain Mom to a gorgeous woman, someone I didn't really know, someone I wasn't allowed to hug or kiss, but could only admire from a distance.

I also remembered my mother's periodic encouragement to me as I moved through my life in jeans and T-shirts. "Wear a little jewelry once in a while," she would urge. "Put on something fancy. It's fun to dress up. It makes you feel like a different person."

I always listened politely but never followed her advice. I was not interested in escaping into glamour—I was into comfort and ease.

But this day, without knowing it, Mom was finally getting her way. That unbidden glitter gave me a splash of glamour. When I arrived at my meeting, I signed in with the receptionist.

"Hey, you look nice," she said, looking carefully at me. "Did you do something different to your hair?"

I shook my head and thanked her. Maybe she saw the silver glints on my face. Maybe she noticed the extra shine on my shirt.

During the meeting, I felt more open and animated. I felt as though I had stepped out of my ordinary clothes and into something more daring and alluring.

When I went to the restroom during a break, I noticed my face still glowed with those little winks of glitter.

Later that afternoon, I went to visit my mother. She sat among the others, ignoring the old Natalie Wood movie on the television. I sat beside her, said her name, and tapped on her arm. On the screen, Natalie Wood was upset with her husband. Mom didn't seem to notice. I put my hand on Mom's red sweatshirt and said, "Hi, Mom."

She looked up and stared at me, like I was a trespasser. Her cold appraisal made me shiver inside. This dowdy, unfriendly woman seemed so far away from the mother I knew.

Then Mom smiled.

"Oh, it's you," she said, although she probably did not know who I was. "La la la," she said and tugged at the sleeve of my turtleneck. She lowered her head and, with shaking fingers, zeroed in on a speck of glitter. She sighed and struggled, trying to pick up that speck. Finally, it stuck on the end of her finger.

"Ha," she said, showing me her fingertip with the silver glint. I wondered if she knew where that glitter was from. I wondered if a spot deep inside her zinged back to a moment when she had stood before her bedroom mirror, admiring herself before she went out.

That night, after a long, relaxing bath, I slipped on my mother's glittery, elegant top. It fit me perfectly. I rummaged in my closet and unearthed the box of costume jewelry Dad had given me when Mom went into the nursing home.

I had never enjoyed jewelry, but now I took out a long, black bead necklace, one Mom used to wear with her black-and-white polka-dotted dress. I slipped on the necklace. Its weight felt comforting along my neck. I felt like I was putting on the lost pieces of my mother. I looked in the mirror and saw that I was shining.

The Very Thought of You

One night, Dad walks into the nursing home's dining room and hears the nurse aides singing "The Very Thought of You."

Dad stands still, transfixed and amazed. This song is significantly different from the rock and roll, metal, or hip-hop usually playing in the dining room.

"Where did you learn that song?" Dad asks, applauding loudly, when the song has ended. He knows from his days as a DJ that Ray Noble composed that song in 1934. He is pretty sure none of the staff were born before the 1960s.

"Jean taught it to us," says Lynell. She gives my mother her last spoonful of butterscotch pudding and points to a woman in a wheelchair at the next table. "You know, Jean used to be a singer when she was younger. We love this song."

"I love it, too," Dad says.

Dad has seen Jean, wheeling slowly through the hallways, but he didn't know she was a singer. That song brings Dad back to his radio days, when he worked the graveyard shift playing such songs. He and Mom went dancing to such big band music and often visited clubs to listen to torch singers breathlessly, tenderly, sadly, lay out such lyrics. This is a song he especially loves.

Often Dad tells me he just doesn't remember things the way he used to. At age eighty-five, he sometimes misplaces words, tucks away the endings to stories in hidden pockets, and forgets what he was going to say. But he happens to remember that Bing Crosby had a big hit with "The Very Thought of You" in 1944. He knows that in 1950 Doris Day sang it in the movie *Young Man with a Horn* and that Rick Nelson sang the song in the 1960s. Nat King Cole, Andy Williams, Rod Stewart, Billie Holiday, Frank Sinatra, and Duke Ellington also sang, played, or recorded that song.

"This song should make a comeback," Dad says to my mother later that evening as he pushes her wheelchair around the nursing home corridors. "It's a timeless song that deserves more attention, don't you think?" He asks Mom the question even though he knows she is staring at her lap, incapable of really listening. "Don't you think this song has the potential to make it big once again?"

She makes a sound that he takes to mean agreement.

"What do you think?" he asks me the next day, when the three of us are eating lunch in the home's private dining room.

"I love the idea," I say, plucking a brownie chunk off my mom's bib. She has been holding onto the spoon, letting the bite of brownie teeter there, making no move to transfer it to her mouth.

"In that case, I have a surprise for you," Dad says. "I have arranged for a special after-lunch concert with Jean."

When our dessert is almost done, Dad goes into the main dining room and comes back minutes later with a solemn-faced Jean.

"Thank you for agreeing to sing for us," I say.

"My voice isn't what it used to be," Jean answers. Then she lowers her head, pauses, and begins to sing. Her voice is low, throaty, and compelling. Her phrasing is fascinating, her sense of style intact, even though some of the notes are blurred.

I have often seen Jean in her wheelchair, parked by the front door of the nursing home, as though she is expecting a taxi or visitor. Like today, she usually wears an unremarkable white sweater and gray sweatpants. Many times, I have said a quick hello as I walk by. She has nodded politely.

But now, I look at Jean more closely. She looks at me as she sings.

I see Jean's elegant cheekbones, hidden under her loose skin. I can imagine how glamorous she would have looked in a clingy black dress, holding the microphone, the spotlight on her, coaxing the audience deeper into the song, the big band backing her up.

Jean doesn't remember much of her big band days: My father gets a few stories from her niece, who visits once a month. What Jean does remember is all the words and the intricate melody to this song, one of the many songs she sang so beautifully during the 1930s and 1940s. She moves gracefully through the lyrics, giving us eye contact, her face soulful and absorbed. Dad looks at Mom to see if she too remembers this old gem. Mom is rolling up the end of her bib. If she notices the music, it is her secret.

Jean finishes and Dad and I applaud. Mom smiles at the sound of the clapping.

"Tell me some of the bands you sang with," I say, eager to know more about this talented woman who must have known how to melt a room. But Jean wheels away. The concert is over and the star doesn't have time to mingle with the audience.

"You can tell how good she was," Dad says. "I was thinking that maybe some of the musicians in town might want to sing that song."

I nod, still thinking about Jean, a woman who has forgotten so much, yet who still remembers this song.

We finish lunch and I take off my mother's bib, brush the extra crumbs off her lap, and wipe the goo off her hands. Then Dad and I maneuver her wheelchair out into the corridor. We stroll through the large dining room, greeting staff and residents, stopping to talk to other visiting family members. Yet even while I am talking, smiling, the lyrics glide through me.

I know what a superb rendition I'd hear in one of our city's great jazz clubs. I also know that this beacon of beauty and hope, this decades-old, aching, heartfelt love song sounds equally beautiful when sung *a capella* in a nursing home in the middle of the afternoon.

An Old-Fashioned Holiday

When I walk through the doors of the nursing home, I find my mother in her wheelchair, right in front of the medication cart, right behind the central nursing station where nurses, delivery people, staff, and family members congregate. Mom is bent over, her baby doll lying across her lap. When I walk up to her, I ratchet up my energy and widen my smile. I am preparing to clown her into a reaction.

Later my father will ask if I think she recognized me.

"No," I will have to tell him. "She did not recognize me. But she did smile."

The smile is important.

My hand waving and head bobbing do their work: Mom does smile, and I can tell she is in her own current version of a good mood. That means she will probably be alert enough at various intervals to smile at me. I am encouraged.

"Music in the dining room," the activity board reads, so I wheel her in that direction. An elderly man with a red-and-white-trimmed Santa hat passes us in the hallway.

"Look, Mom, there's Santa," I tell her.

Having been brought up Jewish, Mom never was all that enthralled with the Claus mythology, and she has not changed.

A young African American man strides by wearing a red Santa hat with black trim.

"There's another Santa," I tell her.

A white-haired woman is in the dining room, busily setting up for the music program. Several patients are already gathered. The woman takes out a microphone, a boom box, an illuminated plastic snowman, and a small silver bell. I continue wheeling Mom down the far corridor, liking the sense of companionship I have from this movement.

As we stroll, a nurse carrying a plate of lettuce walks past us.

"She must have been a good mother," she says, nodding at the way Mom is holding the baby. "She must still be a good mother."

"She is," I say.

I have never really said to my mom, "You were a good mother."

Now I realize she was.

"That's a nice compliment, Mom," I say, leaning down.

I can see that Mom is enjoying the ride. She loved movement when she was younger and was far more adventuresome than Dad when it came to airplanes, ski lifts, fast cars, and speed boats. For her, a biting breeze across the face was thrilling, not threatening. Until she became a mother, that is. Then she abandoned her pleasure in the heights and speed and concentrated on making sure we were slow, safe, and centered.

We roll back into the dining room just as the show is ready to start. The singer, Thelda, kicks off her shoes and presses "play" on the boom box. Above the cheerful sound track, she sings "Jingle Bells." She dances across the room with the remnants of ballroom steps. She stops in front of Mom and sings right to her. She gets on her knees so she can look into Mom's eyes, and keeps singing. Mom notices her and smiles a little.

Thelda moves on, singing to each of the patients gathered around, so intent on making a connection that she often forgets the words.

"Is it all right for your mom to come to Christmas holiday events?" the activity director had asked me when Mom moved into the skilled care section of the nursing home.

"Yes, I'd like her to go to any activities. She likes the extra energy."

I think Mom would approve of my decision, even though she has never celebrated Christmas. Growing up, her immigrant mother held onto the Jewish spirit of her home, kneading dough for Friday evening challah, observing each holiday and prayer period in her own way. Some orthodox women followed the religious law that commanded a small piece of the dough be burned as an offering to God. My grandmother was poor; she did not believe in burning good food, regardless of tradition.

So she sacrificed a portion of the dough to her youngest daughter, my mother Fran. She created a "bread tail," leftover dough that she smeared with butter and sprinkled with sugar and then baked. When Mom used to talk about her mother, she always mentioned this special treat.

Even when I was growing up, and we were the only Jewish family in our neighborhood, my mother still did not sing Christmas songs. She did not willingly go to Christmas parties. She let the holiday rush by her, like a large train whooshing past, ruffling her hair, and leaving her behind.

Now, I am singing Christmas carols to my mom for the first time. She is smiling, though really not at me. But I am sitting beside her while she is smiling, and that makes me happy. She has moved beyond the place where the religions are different, beyond the place where she wants to separate the dough and make a sacrifice for tradition. Her new tradition is anyone who can make her smile.

With each song, from "White Christmas" to "Silver Bells" to "Frosty the Snowman," Thelda moves back to Mom, tapping her, nudging her, shaking a bell almost in her face, acting sillier and sillier. Each time, Mom lifts her head and widens her mouth for a second.

For her finale, Thelda puts on a big red nose and sings "Rudolph." When she dances in front of Mom with that nose, Mom laughs. For several minutes, Mom stays fixated on the scarlet nose, her face a miracle in pure enjoyment. I laugh too, so delighted to see Mom engaged and absorbed. Then, Thelda dances away and Mom's face glazes back over.

Two weeks from now, I will bring a menorah and candles into my mother's room. My father and I will have a short Chanukah ceremony with Mom. She will pick at the shiny paper covering the Chanukah *gelt* (chocolate candy disguised as money). She will slump over in her chair. But she will come back to life when she sees me, her only daughter, wearing a big red nose as I light the menorah.

V.
Celebrating Who She Was:
FEBRUARY TO DECEMBER 2004

Common Grounds

When my parents met in 1948, they had these things in common:
- They were too skinny when they were growing up.
- In early adolescence, they each lost their same-sex parent to cancer.
- They had each been married before—my mother was a widow, my father a divorcé.
- They had served in the army during World War II in England.
- They were dear friends of Bel and Max.
- They were in their thirties and in a hurry to get married and have children.
- They were hardworking and practical.
- They loved their families and wanted to stay connected to them.

During their fifty-plus years of marriage, my parents discovered many new connections and many shared interests, including travel, swimming, walking, listening to jazz, and going to horse races.

During the earliest days of 2004, before my father's sudden death, my parents had these additional things in common:
- Two children, five grandchildren, and one great-grandchild.
- A nursing home staff that admired their love and cared for them.
- A taste for cantaloupe, strawberries, potato soup, and chocolate.
- A sense of humor and the ability to smile even when things were not too funny.

In 1948, when my parents began their correspondence, regular mail cost three cents and airmail cost five cents. My father was a frugal man and he earned a modest income, which he supplemented by occasionally working the ten-dollar window at a nearby racetrack. Yet when writing to my mother, he splurged and sent all his letters by airmail.

On May 14, 1948, he wrote,

> *You ask who are the happy people. I think the happy person is the one who is at peace within himself, who loves and is loved, and the one who lives conservatively but whose life is tempered and savored with a certain amount of abandon and casualness and adventure. And the one who firmly believes in his own God.*

According to this letter, my father died a happy man.

The Missing

People often ask me if Mom knows that her husband died. To answer that question I have to explore the facts and the truth. The facts say that Mom doesn't rationally know anything—she cannot answer a simple question, she cannot recognize me or anyone else by name or context, she does not remember how to put on her shoes or button her blouse. But the truth that goes deep into the soul says yes, she knows. The tops of her knees know and the sides of her cheek know. Her fingertips know and her hair knows. Above all, her heart, which still remembers how to beat, knows that Paul, her husband of fifty-five years, is missing.

My father died suddenly, at age eighty-five. He was playing a solitary game of pool after his supper at the retirement home when he had a massive heart attack and dropped dead. I was out of the country, as far away and inaccessible as I have ever been.

I could not get home for the first days after my father's death, so my daughter Sarah took my father's (and my) place, visiting Mom daily so she wouldn't feel abandoned.

"I didn't tell Nana that Grandpa Pauly died," Sarah tells me when I finally get home. "I thought you would want to do it."

Sarah's words are a cloak of grace for me. I do want to be the one to tell my mother, even though, technically, she won't understand.

What will I say to my mother? How will I communicate with her? I am surprisingly nervous as I walk to her room. Mom is in bed. I sit beside her and stroke her leg through the covers. She glances at me, not registering my presence. I say her name, touch her arm, but I cannot get her attention. Finally, I lower my head to get right into her line of vision, wave my hands wildly, and grin idiotically. Not the greatest warm-up for sharing sad news.

Mom finally laughs at my antics. Then she fades away.

"Mom, I need to tell you something," I begin.

Silently I rehearse the words, filled with the weight of my task. "Dad died. Mom, Dad had a heart attack playing pool and died. Mom, Dad is no longer here, but he still loves you."

But I say nothing.

I cannot tell my mother she will never again see her husband. I cannot say to Frances Barnett that she will no longer have a devoted daily visitor dedicated to her well-being, a man who remembers every good thing about her and adores her just as she is. I cannot stand to think that that part of her life is gone.

I look into her eyes; she looks into mine. *Does she know?* I wonder. *Does she know something is amiss?* I feel that she does.

Then my own grief overwhelms me and I leave.

"I couldn't tell Mom that Dad died," I tell my brother that night over the phone. "It's weird, but I just couldn't make myself do it."

"Take your time," he says.

"Someone has to tell her. I need to tell her. I need to say the words."

"I'm sure she won't mind waiting," Daniel says softly.

Meanwhile, my friends ask, "How is your mom? Does she know? How is she taking it?"

I cannot bear to confess that one whole week after my father's death, I have not yet spoken the words to my mother.

That Saturday, I make myself go to the nursing home again.

Estelle, a patient in assisted living, greets me when I walk in. She is sitting in the reception area with a young woman and a darling baby.

"How's your mom?" Estelle asks, as she always does. "Does she know about your dad? I don't say anything to her. I don't want her to be sad."

I thank Estelle for her kindness. I don't tell her I haven't said anything to my mother either.

I find Mom sitting with a few other residents in front of the video *Field of Dreams.* She appears to be watching the screen, but maybe she is just watching colors and movement.

I wheel her into the reception area so she can see the baby. Mom smiles when she sees the pink-clad little girl.

"What a . . ." she says, and I hear the words without her saying them: ". . . pretty baby." We watch the baby suck on her pacifier, bang a rattle against the chair, and reach out her arms to her mom.

"Baby," Mom says, happily. Then her face falls into something that could be sadness and despair. She looks empty and unfinished. Her dry laugh could easily be the wracking sounds of unformed grief.

I kneel in front of her wheelchair and look into her eyes. She looks back at me and I feel her sadness.

"Mom, Dad died," I say. "That's why he hasn't been here to visit you. You miss Dad, don't you?" I ask.

"Yes," she says, as though she understands my words.

"I miss him too," I say, my eyes filling with tears.

"Yes," she says.

What does she really know? I wonder.

Dad believed Mom knew a lot. He believed she was happy to see him. He had intricate conversations with her and believed her responses, whether silence, nods, or the occasional "Yes, dear," meant something.

I felt skeptical. I saw how randomly Mom responded to me, and I felt Dad was making things up. Now that Dad is dead and I am alone in visiting Mom, I am tempted to believe he was right. I want to believe her sounds and words have meaning.

A man wearing navy-blue pajama bottoms and a red-checked flannel shirt rolls up to the receptionist.

"How are you?" she asks him.

"Not too good," he answers. "I am lost."

"What is your name?" she asks gently.

He spells out his name.

"You live in room 104. Your roommate is Norman," she says.

"Really? I live here? I find that hard to believe," he says.

As I push Mom toward the dining room, I find it hard to believe that she lives here. I cannot believe Dad is dead and I will no longer have someone with whom to discuss Mom's every move and mood. No one else will glory in Mom saying a complete sentence, however short, or reading a word right off the cover of a magazine. No one else will be excited when I report, "Mom laughed."

Mom reaches out to the bright yellow bucket on the cleaning cart. I stop to see if she wants to examine anything else, but her head droops. I take her to the dining room and park her in the usual spot. The terry-cloth bibs are laid out; the kitchen aides are delivering the trays of chicken-fried steak with mashed potatoes.

Usually I feed Mom Saturday lunch, but today, I miss my father too much. I want to get out of here and go home.

I pass the old man with the navy pajamas as I leave.

"I am lost," he tells me.

Yet he keeps going toward the dining room, heading right to his table. Somehow he's going to end up right where he's supposed to be.

Strength in Numbers

"Sometimes the family doesn't want to acknowledge that the patient is dying," Mary, the hospice nurse, tells me as we sit in the nursing home's deserted dining room.

Only two days ago, I learned that my mother, in her advanced Alzheimer's, was eligible for hospice. Only yesterday I called the hospice office, and already my mother has been approved. I listen carefully as Mary explains that a nurse will see Mom twice a week and an aide will visit three times a week. A social worker and chaplain will come once a month. This is the help and support I have been yearning for ever since my father died. Then I realize that Mary just said, "The patient is dying."

An hour ago, I sat in this very dining room and fed the dying woman. She can still open her mouth and take in food. I celebrate this as I see others who can't even do that. She can still watch the food cart go past. Despite her diminished physical self, I never think of my mother as a dying woman, just as a woman who lives in a curiously absent state but still can be amazingly present when the moment is right.

By putting her into the hospice program, am I dooming my mother to only six months to live?

The tabletop is sticky as I sign the papers. I am agreeing my mother will not go to the hospital unless it's absolutely necessary. I am agreeing to take no extraordinary measures. My mother would approve of these decisions, but the finality of them looms large.

I leave the nursing home with a sense of support and sorrow. When my father died, one of the nurses said, "I think your father died because he couldn't stand the thought of your mother dying."

Suddenly, I cannot stand that thought either. Although people look at me with concern and sadness when I tell them my mother has Alzheimer's, I have become used to this strange new connection Mom and I have. I am comforted by the consistency of visiting the nursing home, of seeing my mother, of patiently waiting to see if she will notice me. I like that flash of delight I feel when she finally looks in my direction and takes in my presence, then smiles.

That evening, another hospice nurse calls and discusses taking Mom off her medicines. My throat feels tight as we discuss discontinuing Mom's Alzheimer's medication. Even though I suspect the medication is not working, what if it is? What if I lose Mom's smiles?

"If I notice a difference in her behavior, can we put her back on the medication?" I ask.

The nurse agrees. She understands I may still need the illusion of the medications, even if Mom doesn't.

After our conversation, I sit on my bed and look around me; a *New Yorker* magazine waits to be read, Mom's favorite magazine. A *Gourmet* magazine lies open, a page folded down. It's a chocolate dessert recipe Mom would have loved. On my bedside, I have an enamel pendant my mother made. A friend just sent me some old pictures of my parents, and they are strewn on my bedspread. My mother is so much with me and so far away from me.

The chaplain calls and asks how he can connect spiritually with my mother. I ask him to read psalms and talk to her. I believe the sacred words will go inside and remind her how loved she is.

The next day, the hospice social worker calls. He has been to see Mom and wants to learn more about her. What did she like to do? How can he best communicate with her? I feel myself opening as I describe my mother's literary and artistic nature and suggest ways he can now connect: act silly and make faces to get her attention; take her for a stroll in her wheelchair; read to her; talk to her; show her bright pictures; bring her a baby doll or stuffed toy. He listens attentively and promises to call me in a couple of weeks.

I feel a sense of hope; someone is interested in my mother. She is not just a person who has to be fed, dressed, bathed, and toileted. She is an artist who still likes bright colors, a book lover who likes to hear the sounds of poetry, a woman who enjoys the sound of a man's voice, a grandmother who loves to hold a baby doll.

This interest and attention from others inspires me. I start thinking of more ways I can connect with my mother. I go to fabric stores and buy bright-colored remnants for Mom to see and touch. I collect magazines that feature pictures of animals and children. I listen eagerly when a hospice worker calls to tell me about his or her visit with Mom. This is what I have missed so much since Dad died—people who visit Mom and see her as more than a patient.

I never thought I would say, "Mom has hospice care and I am so happy."

But that's what I am feeling. I tell my brother, my children, my friends.

"I didn't know your mother was dying," a friend responds. "I am so sorry."

But I realize my mother's connection with hospice is nothing to be sorry about. By allowing myself to contemplate and discuss my mother's impending death, I have enriched my life and the life that she has left.

Her husband is dead. Her son lives out of town. Her friends are deceased or infirm. For a while, my mother had only me as a visitor. Now, she has a team, and so do I.

Love Therapy

During the course of Mom's Alzheimer's, she has tried or been subjected to many forms of therapeutic intervention, including physical, recreational, occupational, music, art, and talk therapy. One by one, those therapies slid off Mom without making a mark. My father had to develop his own ways of helping Mom enjoy life despite her diminishing abilities. So he has created love therapy.

He reveals his system to me only once, right before I go on a trip to New Zealand. This is the last time I see my father alive.

"This is the only thing I've found that's still a sure way to get Fran's attention," he told me, and I imagined all the other things he must have tried—singing her a song, trying to amuse her by speaking his leftover childhood Spanish, stroking her hair, telling her jokes, making silly faces, showing her familiar photographs, looking through art books with her, and so many more.

I move closer to see this sure thing. I'm very interested, since I'd had practically no connection with Mom on my last two visits. My dad leans over Mom and gives her a series of rapid little kisses on her cheek. At first, she remains blank-faced. He offers another series and she smiles. Dad gives her the third round of kisses and she laughs.

He smiles at me. "It always works," he says. "The trick is to keep the kisses very light. They surprise her each time."

I am impressed with his technique but too reticent to try it. A series of lovely butterfly kisses from a daughter might not have the same cachet as those from a husband.

After my father dies, I still cannot muster the gumption to try his technique, and I mourn that Mom might have received her last little kisses. But then Pam comes back into our lives. Pam used to work in the Alzheimer's unit and then moved to hospice work.

"You are so pretty, you are so sweet; I just love you so much!" Pam says when she visits, looking at my mother with adoration. Pam reaches out and touches Mom's cheek with such respect and tenderness that I almost cry. How is this woman able to feel such pure, unchecked, enormous love for these patients who have lost so much of themselves? How is she able to feel so joyful, ebullient, and hopeful when she spends time with Mom?

I watch in awe. How simple this form of affection, and yet I have never thought of being so overt and enthusiastic in my love for my mother.

My mother always treated expressions of love with suspicion, like something unlabeled in the back of the freezer. Though I have tried hard to be more open, more affectionate, compared to Pam I am glacial in my reserve.

Did my mother wish I would be more effusive in expressing my love for her? I'd often wished my mother would be more generous and outward in her affection, more able to tell me that she really loved me. Pam shows none of the restraint Mom so carefully modeled for my brother and me. Pam exudes gushiness and enthusiasm in a way I wish I could. I wish I could tell my mother how adorable she is, how marvelous. I wish I could unbutton all my reserve and coo over her, praising her for the extraordinary life she has lived. Only when Mom is silly, giggling, widening her bright smile, can I beam at her with unhampered love. Only when she is curled in her bed, sweet and still as a tired child, staring pensively into my eyes, can I look at her with pure love and acceptance.

I watch Pam carefully as she continues her crooning. Mom is giggling girlishly, adoring the lavish attention, adoring the very behavior she warned us against and tamped down while we were growing up.

By comparison to Pam's praise, my Dad's stream of little kisses seems demure and well behaved. Surely I can manage those. My shyness falls over me as I lean over my mother. Her cheek is soft, and I see a fleck of egg from the morning's meal.

"Lightly." I imagine my father's instructions and skim my lips across her skin. She has no reaction. I try again, making the kissing sound a little louder. A faint smile curves her lips. I try a third time, bringing the kisses close to her eyes. She laughs. My father's technique still works, that one sweet, sure thing.

Words to the Wise

Mom is in bed when I visit one afternoon, her eyes open, her hands twisting the blanket, like a kid who's had enough of her nap. She smiles when I walk in.

"Hi, Mom, how are you?" I say, and think about my friend who decries such pleasantries, thinking they are inane and not designed to inspire a meaningful dialogue. I certainly expect no direct response from Mom, but the greeting makes me feel normal.

"Do you have any?" Mom asks, raising her head.

She looks at me expectantly and I say, "No, I don't have any today."

"How are," she says, and I feel a little thrill at this social nicety.

"I'm fine, Mom. How are you?"

"I know what you mean," she says, staring out toward the hallway.

I am excited by Mom's pointillistic little monologue. Alzheimer's has erased most of Mom's considerable vocabulary, and this spill of words is a treat. As I stroke her arm and smile at her, I realize I am literally listening to my mother's last words.

In the movies, the last words are profound gems of wisdom, uttered upon a deathbed. Those words are a raft to hang onto so you don't drown with grief. Though my mother is lying in bed, she is definitely not dying. In fact, given her immense years and advanced Alzheimer's, she's physically relatively healthy.

"Well we item," Mom says. "All right."

She no longer needs a listener's approval. She no longer checks for understanding. The words spill out, like the random winnings from a nickel slot machine.

"So, but that's," Mom says as I touch her leg.

"Well, we," Mom laughs.

"Why."

"Oh."

"That's right."

Each word is an independent contractor, a one-act play. Mom's words require interpretation, involvement, imagination, and curiosity. Unlike last words in a deathbed scene, Mom's words do not neatly sum up her life or her philosophy. Still, these words are gifts. Many visits have gone by with the barest scraps of language. I get out my pen and paper and write down every one of my mother's last words.

"Okay."

"I don't know."

"I paid."

"But her." Mom points to the blank wall.

"There you are," Mom says, and she may be referring to me.

"Uhuh."

"Yeah."

"I'll try."

As I write, I imagine she is giving me a secret code, sending me a message from the last cognitive bastion of her brain. "I don't know. I paid. I'll try." What depth, what meaning, what spiritual significance these simple phrases might have.

"Since I set up a peg," Mom blurts out. I know she is only partially revealing her intriguing hidden agenda.

Across the hall, a television set blares out the *Jeopardy!* game show theme. The receptionist pages the head nurse. The cleaning cart bumps down the hallway. Two nurse aides walk past, talking about vacation time.

"No," Mom says. She looks right at me and smiles.

"No what, Mom?" I ask.

"But she didn't," Mom says.

As I observe my mom, I listen to the *Jeopardy!* contestants. Their brains are bursting with all kinds of fascinating data. Full, well-formed sentences flow assertively or tentatively from their lips. They are wealthy in concept and language. Mom used to be rich in language, rich from reading, from painting, from going to movies and concerts, from listening to others. She was eager to get into conversations.

I think of times when Mom visited me, and we'd stay up late, drinking coffee, eating cookies, and talking. It was ordinary conversation, unadorned cotton cloth. But now, those casual talks seem like intricate embroidery on plush velvet.

"Where did I get," Mom says.

"You can."

Jan, the activities director, drops in. "Hi, Frances," she croons to Mom. Mom smiles and says, "There just."

"Mom's really talking a lot today," I say.

"She's doing so well," Jan says. I feel a small sense of pride. I have seen my mother praised for many things—for her cooking, her friendship, her gardening, and her oil painting. Today she is being praised for smiling and saying a few words. She is being praised just for being who she is.

Jan looks lovingly at Mom as Mom says, "They don't. Oh really."

"I'm gonna," Mom says after Jan leaves.

"I'm going to leave soon, Mom. I love you, Mom," I say, leaning down to kiss her cheek.

"Yeah, I know that."

I leave quickly, wanting to hang onto that last quartet of words, wanting to believe those words are true and they are just for me.

The Transition

I feel my mother's absence when I walk into the room. Even when her eyes are closed, her lethargy seems beyond sleepiness. Her energy, her spark, is missing.

"Mom?" I say, touching her back. She is curled into an angular fetal position, tight on her side. She does not answer. She does not stir.

I walk down the just-polished hallway to the charge nurse, who reports, "Frances is not eating or drinking."

I call Pam, the hospice nurse.

"It could be a simple virus, a urinary infection, or a small stroke," Pam says quietly. "Or she may be dying. We just have to wait and see."

I sit beside my mother and say, "If you want to stay, I am totally delighted, and if you need to leave, I understand."

I stroke her back, her hair. Her eyelids open and I kneel down so I can look into her eyes. I seem to see a deep sadness. Then her eyelids close.

"I know you miss Dad," I say. I abandon my usual cheerful talk and let the quiet fall between us. Her legs move back and forth, scissoring her knees close to her chest. Her mouth twists. I look closely at her. Is she in pain? How do I read the messages she is sending? How do I help her when the twist of her lips, the fluttering of her hands are the only language I have to go on?

I ask the charge nurse about the medication the doctor preordered, the end-of-life medicine.

"Is she uncomfortable? Does she need that medicine?" I ask, clenching my hands.

The nurse shakes her head. "She'll have a raspy sound and won't be able to breathe. She'll moan. Then she'll need the medicine."

I don't want my mother to moan and have a raspy sound. I sit on the edge of her bed and I wonder if I should stay or leave. If my mother could speak, would I sit at her bedside all day and night? I want to be a good and loyal daughter. Yet part of me wants to rush out into the bright asphalt comfort of the parking lot. *What would my mother do if she were in my position?* I wonder. I take deep breaths and sit beside her for a while longer before I make my escape.

"If my mother were that out of it, I would want her to die," a friend says that evening.

"How can you be sure of that?" I want to ask her.

I think about her words the next afternoon when I visit Mom. I understand what my friend was feeling, but I don't want my mother to die. I am still receiving richness from our relationship, beyond what I thought was possible. I would never have guessed that I could sit on the edge of a hospital bed with a noncommunicative woman and still feel the warmth of connection.

I gently touch my mother's arm. Mom's hair has just been washed, and someone draped a towel around her head and under her chin so she looks like an old-world *baba*. A smiling, blue-suited baby doll on the pillow beside her completes the picture.

Mom is still refusing to eat, one of my favorite nurse aides comes in to tell me.

"I tried to get her to take just a spoonful of potatoes and she spat them right back out," the aide says.

Long ago, my parents told my brother and me they did not want extraordinary lifesaving measures. No breathing apparatus. No forced feeding. Mom has always been strong and opinionated, and even now, when she appears helpless and disconnected, she rejects the unwanted food. I feel a little spark of pride at her determination.

I kneel down, peer between the bed rails, stroke her leg, and look for signs of awareness. Her eyes are closed. She looks peaceful except for the rummaging of one hand under the covers. I touch her covered hand, trying to still her, but she jerks it away.

The next afternoon, I put a book of Mary Oliver poems, a Bible, a bottle of lavender oil, and a picture book of birds into my satchel. I imagine myself soothing Mom with poetry, reading her *Wild Geese* and showing her pictures of birds. But when I see Mom, I want to march right up to the head nurse and demand, "What have you done to my mother?"

Just yesterday, Mom was curled up, breathing like a child with a cold. Now she is on her back, her mouth wide open, her eyes rolled back in her head, oxygen tubes running into her nose. Her breathing is labored, her face gaunt. I feel I am in the presence of death, and I am scared.

I call the hospice, and Pam promises to come by soon. I call Ron and my daughters.

Then, I sit beside Mom and talk to her. I read her psalms and poems. I sing her the Hebrew song she loves and a variety of her favorite show tunes. As I am reading "I will lift up mine eyes into the hills," my daughter Sarah arrives. I know it is hard on her to see her grandmother like this, and I am also immensely grateful for her presence. Pam arrives and instantly starts making Mom more comfortable. She turns off the bright light and removes the oxygen tubes, since Mom is breathing through her mouth. Just Pam's presence makes me more comfortable. Ron arrives and Sarah leaves. Another hospice nurse drops in. Nurses, aides, and kitchen and cleaning staff shyly come in to say good-bye to Mom and to give us hugs. I feel like I am back in my growing-up neighborhood, where the doors were always unlocked and we were always pleased when neighbors dropped in. I feel a sense of pleasure that even to the very end, my mother is loved.

During the next six hours, we simply sit with Mom. Pam and I listen as Mom's breath becomes raspier and there's more time between the breaths. Ron, Pam, and I share stories about life and love, the kinds of stories Mom would enjoy. We read meditations and prayers to Mom. Pam and I have our hands on Mom. Pam kisses her forehead and keeps her comfortable with medication. Ron brings us dinner. Pam's husband drops by, and we invite him to sit with us. Pam has told me her husband is a Muslim and a deeply spiritual person. I feel his compassion when I shake his hand.

I ask if he will share a prayer of transition for Mom. He recites a beautiful Muslim prayer, first in Arabic, then in English. I ask Ron to read the Mary Oliver poem "The Journey."

Mom's breaths become more infrequent. The other sounds in the room fade away. I am holding Mom's hand at the final gentle breath.

I look at Pam and she nods. My mother is dead. I feel elevated and awestruck by the gracefulness of her death. I also cannot believe my mother has actually died. She looks beautiful in an archetypal, haunted way. Her face is like an amazing tribal death mask, and yet she seems peaceful.

I feel both peaceful and numb. When Pam leaves to call the funeral home, I curl up on the bed next to Mom and sob. All the sadness of the last days and weeks wells up inside me, and I wail at the losses. I weep at the thought of being unparented, alone in that primal sense. Then I sit up and keep my hand on Mom's arm until the funeral people arrive.

"My mother is dead." I practice saying the words aloud to see if I really believe them.

Epilogue

Today, my mother's and father's ashes are intermingled in a shared plot in a national veterans' cemetery. They share a headstone, my mother's name and rank—Frances Barnett, Lieutenant—on one side, and my father's—A. Paul Barnett, Chief Petty Officer—on the other. I smile when I see the headstone. Even in death, my mother outranks my father, which is exactly the way he would have wanted it.

After

"Isn't your mom's death a relief?" a friend asks, two months after Mom has passed on. "It must have been so hard seeing her like that."

I understand what my friend is trying to say, but I've been feeling grief, not relief. In the months after my mother's death, my sorrow and sense of loss have surprised me; I thought I'd grieved the loss of my mother during the deepening Alzheimer's process. But I hadn't mourned my new relationship with my less-rational mom, and I am left with sudden tears and vast expanses of mental numbness. Mom was an integral part of my everyday life, and I miss her and the people in the Alzheimer's unit and their caregivers. As a way to work through my loss, I decide to seek new ties with people who have Alzheimer's and additional ways to deepen my understanding of the disease.

I.
Patching Up the Losses:
SEEKING SOLACE AFTER
MOM'S DEATH

Beyond the Diagnosis

I didn't expect to laugh so much, hear such a wealth of spiritual wisdom, or be so uplifted. I didn't expect to meet twenty cheerful and inspiring people at the Early Stage Alzheimer's Support Group.

I attend the group because I want to understand what it is like in the beginning. What is it like to receive and live with a diagnosis of Alzheimer's?

When Mom was diagnosed with dementia, I was too scared, confused, and emotionally involved to think about such questions. The idea of Alzheimer's was initially terrifying to me and to my family.

Even though being around my mom and other people with Alzheimer's had lessened my fear, any time I have one of those "senior" moments of forgetfulness, I instantly worry: Is this normal or is this Alzheimer's?

Now I am in a room with people who have a label to go with their memory loss and lapses. And instead of looking gloomy and stricken, they are laughing.

The facilitator, Michelle, invites people to check in.

"Tell us how you are," she says.

"I lost an uncle this week and I guess I am feeling a little sad," George says. A navy-blue baseball cap shades his cherubic face. In his plaid shirt and jeans, he looks well-worn and comfortable.

"Do people know when you're feeling sad, George?" Michelle asks.

"I don't reckon they do. I don't reckon I like to let on what I'm feeling."

"How many of you let people know when you're sad?" Michelle asks the group.

Several people raise their hands.

"You can see it on my face," one man tells us.

"I had a lesson about sadness when my father died," says Barb, who is new to the group. "A woman came up to me after the funeral and said, 'Aren't you brave, not shedding a tear?' And I thought, 'Aren't I ashamed, not shedding a tear?' I've learned it's important to cry when you're sad."

Barb is sad now because she no longer has a car. She moved here to be closer to her family and finds herself relying on others for transportation.

"I have lost my independence," she laments.

"How many of you think Barbara is an independent woman?" Michelle asks, and many raise their hands.

"She's a clear communicator and very articulate," one woman observes.

"It's not about who's behind the wheel," Michelle tells Barb. "It's about how you see yourself as a person."

"I need to see myself as independent again," Barb says, and everyone nods encouragingly.

Lionel is also unhappy that he can no longer drive. "But it's the right decision. I see things that are not there," he confesses.

The last time she drove, Sherry tells us, she got lost on the freeway. It was so unnerving; she's grateful she no longer has a car.

As Sherry is speaking, Larry walks in.

"Sorry I'm late," he says sheepishly. He is a handsome man in his early fifties. He looks like he'd do a fine two-step in his cowboy boots, western shirt, and jeans. "I got lost. I know where I am, but I don't always know how to get from one place to the other." Just days ago, he says, he got confused in the parking lot of a local mall and had to have a security guard lead him out. He got turned around returning home from a meeting and phoned his wife so she could talk him through the once-familiar streets.

"I know what you mean. My inner maps have disappeared," Louis says. "Now I have to use MapQuest or a city map and really plan how I'm going to get someplace."

Louis, who is in his early sixties and has a PhD, which he says stands for "piled high and deep," does a lot of planning because he has a lot of places to go. He volunteers five days a week at a local charity. He referees soccer games almost every night. He plays bridge. And in the middle of all this he spends an inordinate amount of time looking for "things that were there just a minute ago."

"I function almost normally, but I am not normal," Louis proclaims, and everyone nods. They all know the inner slips and slides that can accost them at any minute.

Around the circle of attendees, people report feelings of both harmony and discord. I remember my mother experiencing such feelings, though she rarely talked about them, and I feel a sense of relief at understanding more deeply some of the emotional dynamics of this disease.

"Some days, time moves along but I don't," says Charlie, who is newly diagnosed and in his mid-fifties. People murmur their understanding.

"I am at peace," Sherry says. Also in her mid-fifties, she is one of the youngest people in her assisted living facility. Her voice is soft, her smile sweet. "I am joyful and hopeful."

Dick, a former attorney, says he feels better now that he is back to playing tennis. "Then some days, I'm out of it." He shakes his head. "Well, I just have to laugh."

"That's what I do; I laugh at Alzheimer's," Louis says.

"I am a positive person," Bob, one of the newer group members, reports. "I like to have a lot of experiences, and this is one of life's experiences."

I planned to take notes, but I am too absorbed. This group is embodying some of the more meaningful messages I have heard from therapists and read in self-help books. Their sense of hope and optimism in a situation that would daunt many people reminds me that anything is possible.

"I wish people knew that Alzheimer's is not like it used to be," Lois says. She looks elegant with her beautiful white hair and her stylish pink pants suit. "It's not just a death sentence. I was astounded when I first came to this group. I couldn't believe how upbeat and encouraging everyone was."

Michelle asks the group what kinds of messages she should put on the signs for them to carry at an upcoming Memory Walk fund-raising event.

"We never give up!" Sherry says.

"We're still the same," someone else suggests.

"You must have hope."

"We have Alzheimer's, not leprosy," Bob offers, and everyone cheers.

The group ends. The caregivers' group, which was meeting in the next room, also ends, and family members reunite.

Lois offers me a beaded bracelet that she made. Sherry reaches out her hand and thanks me for coming. I feel exhilarated as I walk to my car. I had expected to attend a group glumly talking about coping with a dreaded disease. Instead I encounter a group of people determined to embrace their new challenges and live life to the fullest.

The Hills Are Alive

My mother's passion for painting inspires me to attend a Memories in the Making art class, designed for people who have Alzheimer's. I want to meet some of the artists and feel my connection to Mom through the artistic process. Still, I feel nervous as I walk through the nursing home and into a small activity area.

"We have a visitor today," Harriet, the facilitator, tells the assembled group.

Everyone looks up.

"Wonderful," says one woman.

"Come paint with us," says another.

I smile and begin to relax. Harriet hands me bowl of water, paper, brush, and watercolors and finds me a place between Norman and Margaret. Then Harriet introduces me to the artists at work.

Ed, a former veterinarian, has a photograph of a great blue heron in front him. He is a slight, spry man who looks like he could fix any emergency.

"That bird is really coming along," Harriet tells Ed. Using colored pencils, he has sketched the upper half of the heron. The bird has an inquisitive appearance.

Now Ed is concentrating on drawing an assortment of cattails, reeds, and other marsh plants in the background.

"Ed is married to Rhea," Harriet tells me as I look at the splash of free-form color on Rhea's page. Rhea, who also has Alzheimer's, is creating a sunset with vivid oranges and purples. I smile at the difference in their art—Ed's controlled sense of detail, Rhea's spontaneous bursts of color. I imagine those traits made for a good partnership.

"We've been together twenty-two years," Rhea says. She is plump, with a welcoming air.

"Or maybe it's twenty-five years. Do you remember?" she asks Ed.

"A long time," Ed says.

At the head of the table, Betsy grins as she shows me a penciled caricature of a kitty cat. The cat's mischievous expression is similar to Betsy's. "It's not quite right, but I'm working on it," she says.

Evelyn has a shy, solemn manner. She holds a small photo of a cardinal and looks at the blank white paper in front of her, as if the relationship between paint and paper is sheer mystery. Her smile is full of apology. "And they were friends," she says when I introduce myself. "And nice to me and my geranium."

Margaret has a photograph of fence posts and her penciled sketch of four posts.

"Something is wrong," Margaret tells us.

"There are five posts in the photo," Harriet tells her. "But you can have four if you like."

"No, I want it right," Margaret says. She picks up a ruler and begins to insert an extra post.

"You must be an organized person," I say, admiring the methodical way she analyzes the posts. "Yes," she says. "I went to college in Michigan and then my daughter went to college in Indiana. Now she lives in Indiana, I think."

Norman has beautiful silver hair and deep brown eyes, and is dressed in a polo shirt and slacks. He looks like he could easily be running a meeting or entertaining important clients on the golf course. Formerly an engineer, he was living in New Orleans, Harriet explains, and was moved up here to be near family. He is recreating a mountain lake scene and has quickly captured the essence of his photograph.

"I just use my fingers to gauge the perspective," he tells me when I compliment his work. In his spare time, Harriet says, he is recreating maps of area bridges.

As I sit down to my own paper and watercolors, I hear someone from the room next door singing melodies and lyrics I recognize as being from *The Sound of Music.*

"Music and art," I say. "What a wonderful combination."

"We all like to sing, don't we?" Harriet says and begins singing her own version of the song. Ed, Rhea, Betsy, and Margaret join in. Norman concentrates on shading the mountainsides a shadowy purple.

Then Harriet begins singing "She'll Be Coming Around the Mountain" while she walks around, admiring people's art and asking if they need fresh water or help. As I moisten my watercolors and stretch purple waves across my paper, I feel a sense of comfort and connection. Harriet knows how to create a space where the artist can blossom.

"Ed and I have three children, and two of them are ministers," Rhea says.

"My daughter lives in Michigan," Margaret says. "I went to college in Michigan."

"I didn't go to college," Rhea says a little sadly. "My dad was real strict. I left home when I was eighteen and got married and started having babies. We have three children, and two of them are ministers. We had a minister at our wedding and Ed sang 'Always' to me." Ed smiles shyly and begins to sing the song. Everyone joins at the last word, "always."

Rhea dabs at her eyes.

I spread more color across my paper, blues and purples, as Rhea describes Thanksgiving dinner at her son's house, "Fried turkey and grits on china plates," she says.

Harriet starts a verse of "Over There," and everyone joins in.

"It's almost time to stop for today," Harriet says. I glance at my paper, a blur of color, with no figures to disturb its purity. I take a final walk around the table. Margaret has added a horizon line to the fence row. Evelyn's paper is still blank, and she smiles without looking away from the photograph of the cardinal. Betsy's sassy kitty is now contemplating a merry little mouse. Ed's heron looks ready to win an Audubon competition. Rhea's sunset is colorful and dramatic. Norman's hills look complete, and his lake is taking shape. My own painting seems plain and unsophisticated next to the rest of the art.

"Have any of these people had art lessons before?" I ask as I help Harriet empty water bowls and clear away used paper towels.

"No," she tells me.

For most of these artists, this is a tender and uncertain time in their lives, a time when memory and rational thinking are often blotchy and blurred, where words can fall away as quickly as autumn leaves. Designed by the Alzheimer's Association, this art program gives them a chance to express themselves freely and creatively. Out of the mental chaos and confusion, the art emerges, vibrant, true, and exciting.

As I am taking leave of Harriet, Norman comes back into the room.

"Is there white?" he says.

"What do you mean?" Harriet asks.

"I'm going to need white for the snow on the mountaintops," Norman says. "I wondered if you had any white."

"I'll be sure I have some for next time," Harriet promises. "Meanwhile, would you like one of these white pencils?"

Norman takes the pencil. "There has to be snow," he tells me. "That makes all the difference." His walk is steady and sure and he leaves the room, softly humming. I recognize the song. "The Hills Are Alive." Alive.

The Circle of Memories

I am not prepared for the rush of emotions I feel when I walk into the nursing home. Instantly, I see a woman who reminds me of my mother, with her curly white hair and sweet, vacuous stare. I have not been inside a nursing center since Mom died, but my friend Scott has invited me to visit his facility and be part of his validation circle, and I am curious.

Months earlier I had met Naomi Feil, who founded validation therapy. Her techniques help caregivers authenticate the emotions and communications of people who have Alzheimer's. Scott is a trained validation facilitator and uses the circle as a way to honor, inspire, encourage, and connect people.

In the small meeting room, Scott intersperses the people who are willing communicators with people who have more difficulty speaking.

Margaret sits on one side of me. Scott brings in Irene, who settles on my other side. Irene wears a bright pink top with bunnies on it, white pull-on slacks, a cranberry-colored glass-bead necklace, and a large rhinestone ring. She takes one look at me and announces, "I don't know you."

I introduce myself. Instantly, she takes my hand and holds it. Just as instantly, I fall in love with her. During the last years of my mother's life, Mom and I did a lot of hand-holding, and I miss that simple yet deep connection. This is the way to begin a friendship, I think.

Today's group happens to be all female. Scott invites Irene and another woman to be song leaders and, shyly, Irene agrees, saying, "I don't really know any songs." Scott begins singing "I've Been Working on the Railroad." Slowly, Irene and everyone else join in.

As part of the opening ritual, Scott asks another woman to welcome us. At first, this small woman, hunched over in her wheelchair, is silent, and I wonder if she can speak. I bite my lip as she fights to form and say the words. "I want to welcome each of you to this gracious gathering." I think about my usual impatience; if I had not been sitting in this circle, I might have missed this woman's words and the glow that fills her face when she finishes speaking.

We go around the circle and introduce ourselves. In some meetings this may be a routine activity, but here it is a ritual mixed with tension and imagination. Edna Lou can't remember her name, but she has ideas. "It's dog, mud, it's a drunk going around. You can call me honey. Honey," she concludes.

I silently root for Sarah as she contemplates the question of her name for a while before producing both her name and an address.

Ellen is flustered. I worry as she ponders and nothing comes to her. Scott offers, "Is your name Ellen?" A lovely smile accompanies her grateful nod.

As Scott moves around the circle, each person receives attention from the group. I feel the power and pleasure of that attention when it is my turn to say, "I am Deborah, from Kansas City." The women nod and murmur as if I have said something important.

As I watch and listen, I realize I am in a circle with an amazing variety of women: women who brim with wit and mischief, women of prayer and serenity, women of secret smiles and silent musings, and women who love to help and serve. Scott honors and includes each person in whatever way is right for her.

We sing another song and Fanny says, "I thought I was crazy once, but it was all in my mind." As we laugh, Fanny advises, "You should laugh a lot every day."

I remember a childhood birthday party, with a circle of children all clustered around a piñata. Inside this ordinary papier-mâché animal were treats and prizes. Instead of using sticks, we poked gingerly with pencils, trying to work through the thick layers to get to the luscious sweets. This validation circle is doing the same thing.

Margaret says, "I love you all and I will always be there for you." I gently squeeze Irene's hand, and she smiles at me.

As the meeting ends, Scott kneels before each woman, saying her name and thanking her for coming. I watch, awestruck, as he patiently moves around the circle, each woman flowering under the attention. When he says to me, "Deborah, thank you for coming to this meeting and thank you for being part of it," I feel an odd sense of pleasure and achievement. In all the many meetings I have attended, no one had ever knelt in front of me and thanked me for showing up.

The nurse aides come in to help people back to their rooms.

"I loved meeting you," I say to Irene, reluctantly letting go of her hand.

"Come back," she says.

"I will."

I know I will return, but not just because of my interest in people who have Alzheimer's. I will return because of the wonderful connection I felt, sitting quietly in a circle of welcoming people, sharing old songs, saying our names, and feeling honored and validated simply for being.

II. Taking Care of Yourself: A Caregiver's Guide

I walk out of the Alzheimer's unit with my head buzzing, my hands trembling; I lean against a wall in the lobby, feeling sad, confused, and terrified. I have suddenly realized that if illness can take hold of my mother, it can take hold of me. I take a deep breath and shove my hands into my pockets, eager to find my car keys and drive away from this place.

But my car keys are not there; I search my purse. No car keys. I scour my pockets—no keys. I can't believe I am already losing my mind! I can barely breathe as I run to my car, praying that somehow I left my keys in the ignition. The car is unlocked, but the keys are not inside; they are not on the seat and not on the floor.

Then I knock into something with my foot. I look down at the parking lot; there are the keys, half hidden under the car. Relief floods me as I pick them up and settle into the car. It hasn't happened to me, not yet, at least.

I quickly learned that fear of impending dementia was common among Alzheimer's caregivers. I also learned to expect I would more frequently lose or misplace something after being with my mom.

During my journey with Mom, I was always looking for ways to soothe my fears and focus on blessings, teachings, and gifts. I sought ideas that would calm and nurture me. Here are some of the simple tips that helped me; I gathered them from my own experiences, from other caregivers, and from experts in the field.

Staying Connected and Making the Most of Your Time Together

For many families, Alzheimer's seems like an ending. But it can be the beginning of a deep emotional and spiritual experience. As you move through the initial feelings of fear and confusion, I encourage you to look for the gifts and blessings in the caregiving journey. Here are some simple tips for staying connected:

- Celebrate the person who is still with you. Instead of comparing the person with Alzheimer's to his or her earlier self, you may notice a different, but still interesting, person.
- Journey into his or her reality. If Mom (or Dad or spouse) talks about going home, ask questions to learn what home means to him or her *now*. When you enter the world of the person who has Alzheimer's, you may find humor, insight, and some fascinating details.
- Explore ways to communicate other than talking. Look through photo albums together. When you visit, bring a goody bag of different objects to touch and talk about. Read poetry aloud. Sing old songs. Put together scrapbooks. Go for walks. Hold hands. Gaze into each other's eyes. Connect through tender touch.
- Savor and write down the stories you're told, even if you hear certain stories again and again. When you write down the most often-repeated stories, you create a legacy to share with family, friends, and other caregivers.

- Share your experiences with friends and family, and accept their support. Telling your own stories helps you articulate and notice the gifts in your caregiving journey.
- Ask friends and family for their own stories about the person with Alzheimer's; this helps them stay involved and reminds them to stay connected with you all.

Journaling and Blogging: Sharing Your Own Stories

Journaling on my experiences with my mom and Alzheimer's was a deep blessing. Using the art of rapid writing, where I poured out my experiences without worrying about spelling, punctuation, or grammar, deeply enriched my journey.

Here are some reasons to journal or blog:

- The writing process can help you define, express, and eventually release your natural anger, fears, and confusion.
- When you record your experiences, you're also honoring the person with Alzheimer's for the way he or she is handling the disease. I didn't realize how courageous my mother was until I went back and read of my encounters with her.
- Writing about your experiences gives you immediate release; reading what you've written offers you a wider picture, allowing you to notice what you've learned and experienced.

Here are some tips for encouraging the writing process:

- Keep a notepad handy, so you won't forget your person's unexpected bits of wisdom.
- Don't judge yourself or your writing. You're simply acting as a reporter, noting the facts of this new world.
- Find a safe place to store your writing until you are ready to read it.

- Give yourself a treat and share snippets of your work with others. You are not alone in what you are going through; by reading your experiences aloud you give others a sense of connection and empathy, and you help decrease your own sense of isolation.

Activating Your Advocacy

Just by sharing your caregiving stories, you are being an advocate for people who have Alzheimer's. Other simple acts of advocacy include these:

- Ask other caregivers what they're doing to help bring attention to the issues of Alzheimer's.
- Tell other people what your family is going through; describe the physical, emotional, and financial impact. If they ask how they can help, graciously accept the offer and give them something specific they can do.
- Memorize a few simple statistics about Alzheimer's to share when the time is right.
- Attend support meetings or other Alzheimer's-related events, or host such an event.
- Help families living with Alzheimer's by staying connected with them; visit them or invite them to visit you. Encourage them to share their stories.
- Join an advocacy team, such as one from the Alzheimer's Association, and become aware of pending Alzheimer's-related legislation.
- Write or call your political representatives, letting them know the importance of increasing Alzheimer's research funding.

Need some facts to activate your advocacy?

- The number of Americans living with Alzheimer's disease is 5.4 million.

- One in eight older Americans has Alzheimer's disease.
- Alzheimer's disease is the sixth-leading cause of death in the United States and the only cause of death among the top ten in the United States that cannot be prevented, cured, or even slowed.
- More than fifteen million Americans provide unpaid care valued at $210 billion for persons with Alzheimer's and other dementias.
- Worldwide there are 7.7 million new cases of Alzheimer's every year.

Visit www.alz.org or www.alz.co.uk for more information.

Connecting Through the HERO Project

My partner Ron and I started the HERO Project because we wanted to help people with dementia stay connected with their families and friends. The HERO Project combines storytelling and scrapbooking techniques in a dynamic, playful, and interactive process that highlights and celebrates everyday events and honors the person who has Alzheimer's.

You can do HERO Projects at home or in a care facility and include people of all ages and abilities. HEROES are invited to talk about their lives, help write a personal story, pose for photographs, and be part of putting together a collage. The result is a visual and lasting memory, something to read through again and again.

This project invites:

- Self-esteem
- Creativity
- Connection
- Capturing of personal or group history
- Celebration of personal quirks and qualities

For us, doing these HERO Projects gives us a chance to come together to honor and celebrate a person (or a group of people) who might not feel heroic right now or might love receiving a little extra attention.

The ten steps for creating a HERO Project are simple and as interactive as you want them to be.

1. Select a HERO or HEROES to star in the story. There are at least two types of stories: one that focuses on a singular HERO and has a supporting cast, and one that is an ensemble story with a lot of HEROES.

2. Brainstorm. Discuss the likes and dislikes, qualities, or life events
    for the HERO that might make an interesting story line. Involve
    as many people as you like. Share some memories; ask, what are
    characteristics we should highlight in the story? Are there favorite
    sayings or memories we should include?

3. Create the storyline. Base your story on the HERO's
    characteristics, such as bravery or curiosity. Creating the storyline
    gives you a chance to talk about the person's hobbies, preferences,
    likes, and dislikes. This reminds you that there is a long life behind
    this person full of adventures, trials, triumphs, and stories. You can
    use a simple template:

    - What does the HERO want?
    - What gets in his or her way?
    - How does he or she overcome the challenge?

4. Share the storyline with the participants.
    In some settings, the people or groups of people may not be able
    to contribute to or react to the storyline. You can simply tell them
    about the storyline on the day of the photo shoot. (See number
    five, below.)

5. Have a photo session or sessions. Involve as many people as you like,
    taking plenty of photos to illustrate the storyline.

6. Print the best photos. We take a lot of digital photos to make sure
    we have enough good shots.

7. Print the storyline—and be ready to make changes in it as
    necessary. It is not necessary to have access to a computer printer;
    you can also handwrite the story.

8. Gather the group once more for a creative "story-scrapping"
    session. You'll want colored paper for the background(s), magazines
    for additional photos or quotes, glue, scissors, and tape. Let people

look through magazines, tear, cut, and paste. You can also include personal photographs, favorite sayings, and more.

9. Share the finished story by reading it aloud and sharing the pictures.

10. Make copies as needed for HEROES and supporting casts and families, or send the book via email.

Using HERO Projects as a Family

Here's an example of our first HERO Project, which began as a way to help connect my ten-year-old nephew Jake with his grandmother, who then was in the early stages of Alzheimer's. We illustrated our script with photos and enhanced it with pictures and quotes from magazines.

The Education of Jake the Strong: Power Isn't Everything

Once upon a time there was a boy named Jake who was very strong.

He was so strong because he lifted weights and ran a mile every day.

He punched boxing bags.

He was so strong he could move cars. He could topple over giant water towers.

He was so strong he could move just about anything.

Except Nana.

He tried pushing.

He tried pulling.

He tried lifting.

Nothing worked.

He thought and thought and finally decided to consult a wise old man, his grandfather Pauly.

"Pauly, how can I move Nana?" asked Jake.

"Easy," said Pauly. "Nana, come here, please."

Nana moved to Pauly and gave him a big hug.

And the strongest kid in the world learned there is at least one thing stronger than power: love.

This was a healing project for my family. Jake and I worked on the script, and then shared it with my parents. We all did the photo shoots together. My mother was going through a stage of being very resistant, and she had a good time acting out her resistance. My dad, who was pretty depressed by all that was going on with my mom, actually smiled and laughed during the process. Once we developed the pictures, we all sat around the table and put the book together. Jacob wrote out the script. Mom and Dad enjoyed leafing through magazines for sayings and ideas. Most of all, they enjoyed sitting around with us with something to focus on other than Mom's Alzheimer's, and they loved the finished product. We each related to the message, and we shared the scrapbook with our friends and relatives.

Sharing this story inspired people to reach out to my parents and stay connected.

Using a HERO Project in a Care Center

We created a HERO Project for Ron's father Frank when he moved into assisted living. We sailed through Frank's life story, using the theme "Lucky Frank"; this is a quality that Frank had all his life—luck, and the ability to appreciate it.

We shared the finished product with Frank, with the staff, and with our out-of-town family via email. We used parts of the scrapbook along with other familiar photos in a memory box outside Frank's room.

When Frank had to move from assisted living into an Alzheimer's unit, we used "Lucky Frank" to introduce Frank to all the staff. The book stayed in Frank's room, and we often used it to jump-start a visit. Frank enjoyed looking at the book every time. Often we read the book out loud, and sometimes he read along. This simple book gave us all, particularly Frank, a lot of pleasure. It helped us celebrate his past and honor him in the present.

For more ideas about the HERO Project, please visit our website: www.thecreativityconnection.com.

Resources

Here are resources to help you further your connections and support.

Organizations
National Alzheimer's Association
www.alz.org
24-hour help line, 800-272-3900
The National Alzheimer's Association offers a wealth of information and support. The staff at your local Alzheimer's Association can guide you to myriad resources, from support groups to Alzheimer's facilities to day care and memory care programs. Their goal is to educate and support.

Alzheimer's Foundation of America
www.alzfdn.org
866-232-8484
Their mission is to provide optimal care and services to individuals confronting dementia, and to their caregivers and families, through member organizations dedicated to improving quality of life.

Caregiver Action Network
www.thefamilycaregiver.org
800-896-3650
The Caregiver Action Network (National Family Caregivers Association) educates, supports, empowers, and speaks up for the more than sixty-five million Americans who care for loved ones with a chronic illness or disability or the frailties of old age.

Overseas

www.**dementiacareaustralia**.com

www.**dementiafoundation**.org.au

www.**cecd-society**.org

Suggested Reading

Bell, Virginia, and David Troxel. *A Dignified Life, Revised and Expanded: The Best Friends™ Approach to Alzheimer's Care: A Guide for Care Partners.* Baltimore, MD: Health Communications, Inc., 2012.

Brackey, Jolene. *Creating Moments of Joy: A Journal for Caregivers.* Jolene Brackey, 2007.

Callone, Patricia R., Connie Kudlacek, Barbara Vasiloff, Janaan Manternach, and Roger Brumback. *A Caregiver's Guide to Alzheimer's Disease: 300 Tips for Making Life Easier.* New York: Demos Medical Publishing LLC, 2006.

Doraiswamy, P. Murali, and Lisa P. Gwyther. *The Alzheimer's Action Plan: What You Need to Know—and What You Can Do—About Memory Problems, from Prevention to Early Intervention and Care.* New York: St. Martin's Griffin, 2008.

Genova, Lisa. *Still Alice.* New York: Pocket Books, a division of Simon & Schuster, Inc., 2007, 2009.

Kuhn, Daniel, and Jane Verity. *The Art of Dementia Care.* Independence, KY: Delmar Cengage Learning, 2008.

Lee, Hilary, and Trevor Adams. *Creative Approaches in Dementia Care.* Basingstoke (UK): Palgrave MacMillan, 2011.

Mace, Nancy, and Peter Rabins. *The 36-Hour Day: A Family Guide to Caring for People Who Have Alzheimer Disease, Related Dementias, and Memory Loss.* Baltimore, MD: Warner Books Edition, Johns Hopkins University Press, 1999.

McCurry, Susan. *When a Family Member Has Dementia: Steps to Becoming a Resilient Caregiver.* Westport, CT: Praeger, 2006.

Stankard, Bernadette, and Amy Viets. *Dancing in the Dark: How to Take Care of Yourself When Someone You Love Is Depressed.* Las Vegas, NV: Central Recovery Press, 2011.

Credits

Some of the stories in this collection were previously published.

"A Drop of Honey," *The Washington Post*. September 22, 2003.

"Let It Be," *Woman's Day*. May 16, 1998.

"In the Eyes of the Beholders," *Chicken Soup for Every Mom's Soul*. February 14, 2005.

"Love in the Land of Dementia," *Chicken Soup for the Caregiver's Soul*, 2012, and in *Spirituality & Health*.

About the Author

Deborah Shouse is dedicated to celebrating love in all its glorious guises. She is a writer, speaker, editor, and creativity catalyst. Her writing has appeared in periodicals such as the *Washington Post, Reader's Digest, Newsweek,* and *Woman's Day.* Deborah has been featured in many anthologies, including dozens of *Chicken Soup* books. Deborah also writes a weekly column on love for the *Kansas City Star* and cofacilitates the Kansas City Writers Group.

Deborah has worked with companies such as Hallmark Cards, Stowers Innovations, and Ascension Health. She has authored a number of business books and is the coauthor of *Antiquing for Dummies, Yes You Can! Raise Financially Aware Children,* and *Entrepreneurs + Mentors = SUCCESS.*

Deborah and her partner Ron Zoglin are passionate advocates for caregivers and for people who have Alzheimer's. They have performed Deborah's writings for Alzheimer's associations and caregiver groups in the United States, New Zealand, Nova Scotia, Puerto Rico, England, Ireland, Italy, Turkey, Chile, and the U.S. Virgin Islands. At every encounter with caregivers, Deborah learns more about the incredible power of love.